Praise for Descent into Dementialand

Biography & Memoir Finalist, 2025 Maxy Awards

"Four and a half stars. Very highly recommended, but be ready to explore every emotion you have; it's the least the author deserves."
— Matt McAvoy, Author/Editor

"Sherry Hobbs's third book, Descent into Dementialand, is a heartfelt memoir chronicling a relationship of enduring love and resilience in the face of her husband, Mike's, battle with dementia—Logopenic Progressive Aphasia. From a picture-perfect marriage to a heartbreaking diagnosis seemingly triggered by a family tragedy, Sherry shoulders immense responsibility while clinging to their unbreakable bond. With wry humor and the author's glass-half-full approach, this book had me flipping pages, even though I knew Mike's disease promised no happy ending. I finished this book in two days—I couldn't stop reading about Sherry's love for Mike and the ways Mike reciprocated even as his condition deteriorated. A must-read!"
— Cam Torrens, Award-Winning Author

Descent into Dementialand is sometimes terrifying but always brutally honest and beautifully recounted. In her tour de force, the author, Sherry Hobbs, opens the door to the struggles she and her husband, Mike, endure while he disappears from within, due to Logopenic Progressive Aphasia, a type of dementia. She tells the story with fearlessness, unbridled love, and kindness. A powerful book—five stars could never measure the quality of her writing nor the impact this work will have on her readers. Bravo, Sherry Hobbs!"

— Christopher Amato, Author, Peace River Village, Shadow Investigation

"Sherry Hobbs's latest memoir, Descent into Dementialand, is a touching and heart-wrenching tribute to her dear husband diagnosed with a rare form of dementia. In the early stages of the disease, it may be easy to make excuses for the subtle symptoms that were appearing, but as the years go on, a diagnosis seems inevitable. Living with a person who is in cognitive decline is not an easy thing to do. Hobbs makes no apologies for the difficult range of emotions she feels as she embarks on this most unwelcome journey. She unabashedly shows readers that caring for a loved one with this disease does not automatically turn a person into a saint. With love, compassion, and a sprinkle of humor, Sherry Hobbs gives us a glimpse into the secret lives of those with dementia and those who love them. This book can, and should, speak to anyone caring for a loved one, not just those with dementia. She gently shows us that this new journey into an uncertain future can be filled with small victories by simply looking to the past. Learning to live in the moment is a skill we should all strive for—we have so much to learn from her husband, Mike, and his dog."

— Lisa Febre, Award-Winning Author of Round the Twist and Welcome to the Bright

DESCENT
INTO
DEMENTIALAND

Sherry Hobbs

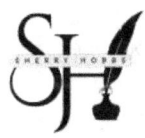

ISBN 13 Paperback: 979-8-99-851280-3

ISBN 13 Ebook: 979-8-99-851281-0

ISBN 13 Hardback: 979-8-9985128-2-7

Library of Congress Control Number: 2025906220

Cover design: Victoria Kaer, DarkAngelGraphics
Interior design: Elaine Aucoin Schroller, elaineschroller.com

All photos: Courtesy of the Hobbs family
Brain Function and MRI illustrations: Shutterstock; Brain icon: BookBrush

v.04282025

Contents

This book is dedicated to all who care or have cared for loved ones with dementia. It is a long journey requiring great patience, flexibility, and sacrifice. I cannot think of many things one can do for another person that are more important or show greater love than to provide safety, security, and the opportunity to help someone live out the rest of their lives with respect, dignity, independence, and joy. I hope that hearing about our journey will inspire and inform.

If you find it helpful, please share it as widely as possible. The profits from this book will go to Alzheimer's and dementia research in the hope that a cure can be found.

Cure Alzheimer's Fund https://curealz.org/
100% of donations go to support research

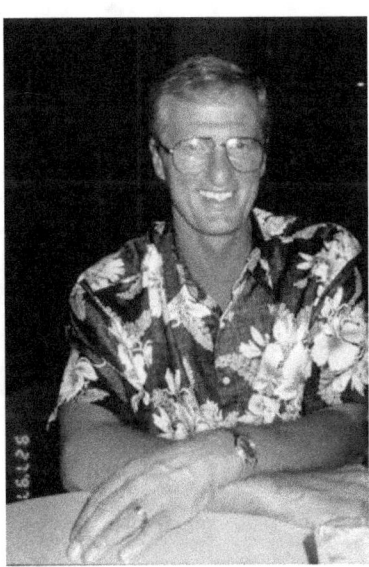

Mike, always my Prince Charming

All the world's a stage,
And all the men and women merely players;
They have their exits and their entrances;
And one man in his time plays many parts,
His acts being seven ages ...

... Last scene of all,
That ends this strange, eventful history,
Is second childishness and mere oblivion;
Sans teeth, sans eyes, sans taste, sans everything.

— William Shakespeare
from As You Like It

ACT ONE
Normaland and Dementialand

Throughout the book, charts like the one below will appear at the beginning of some scenes. Showing typical behaviors at each stage will help the reader follow the progression of Mike's dementia.

Stages 1-4 - Global Deterioration Scale (GDS) / Reisberg Scale

Diagnosis	Stage	Signs and Symptoms	Expected Duration of Stage
No Dementia	Stage 1: No Cognitive Decline	– Normal function – No memory loss – People with NO dementia are considered in Stage 1.	Hopefully forever!
Pre-dementia	Stage 2: Very Mild Cognitive Decline	– Forgets names – Misplaces familiar objects – Symptoms not evident to loved ones or doctors	Unknown. Very common.
Pre-dementia	Stage 3: Mild Cognitive Decline	– Increased forgetfulness – Slight difficulty concentrating – Decreased work performance – Gets lost more frequently – Difficulty finding right words – Loved ones begin to notice	The average duration of this stage is between 2 years and 7 years.
Early-stage	Stage 4: Moderate Cognitive Decline	– Difficulty concentrating – Forgets recent events – Cannot manage finances – Cannot travel alone to new places – Difficulty completing tasks – In denial about symptoms – Socialization problems: Withdraws from friends or family – Physician can detect cognitive problems	The average duration of this stage is 2 years.

Stages 1-4 Table: Applicable to Scenes 4 through 21

geriatric-resources.com/html/gds.html

Introduction
Two Worlds on Planet Earth

Once upon a time, *a lovely, young princess lived in a land not very far away called Normaland. Although not beautiful, she had long eyelashes, clear skin, a pretty smile, straight, white teeth the tooth fairy (and her orthodontist) had bestowed upon her... and good hair, or so her hairdresser told her.*

One day, after kissing several frogs, the princess met a prince. He was tall, handsome, and intelligent. And he made her laugh. Soon, they fell in love. She held his hand, looked into his eyes, and said, "We are partners and are going to have grand and glorious adventures on this incredible voyage called life." And so they began their expedition through Normaland.

The princess was right. Blessed by her fairy godmother, the couple had marvelous adventures throughout the universe, avoiding as many black holes as they could see for the next forty years. A black hole has a great effect on the fate and circumstances of an object crossing it. The boundary of no escape is called the event horizon.[1]

However, one day, they stepped into an enormous black hole that threatened to consume them, but they eventually clawed their way out and kept moving forward along the path, step by step. After traveling only a few feet, they encountered a large, ugly, hairy ogre who introduced himself as Sir Ratt. "Oh, pray tell, sir, we're looking to avoid another black hole on the voyage of life adventures," the princess said. "We have heard of a treacherous park called Dementialand, which we want to avoid. Is there a sign that leads

---

1. Hamilton, A. "Journey into a Schwarzschild Black Hole." *jila.colorado.edu*

us away? Is there a yellow brick road pointing in the other direction we could follow?"

Ratt made a toothy, ragged grimace. "Dementialand?" he snarled through his broken teeth. "There are no signs at all. Just keep walking. The black hole is invisible. You have to hope not to stand on the edge because you will find yourself at the event horizon, and there is no escape from Dementialand if you do."

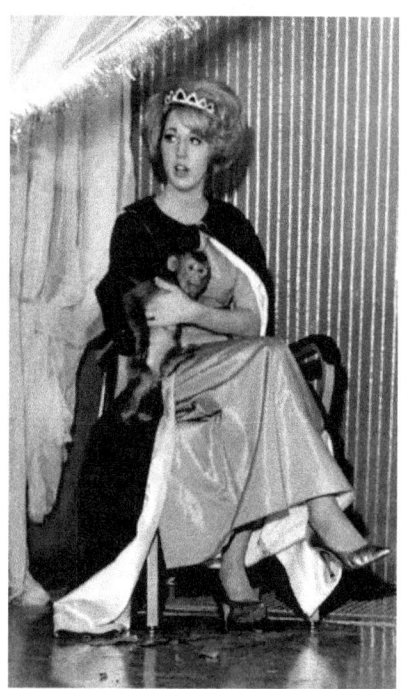

The princess at 19

Scene 1

The Slippery Slide into FrontierWorld

Once upon a time, Mike and I lived blissfully in Normaland, where most people on Earth live. We both had successful careers and a beautiful, brilliant, yet troubled son. We'd traveled extensively, skied frequently for six months of the year, and golfed weekly at beautiful country clubs in Southern California all year round. It was a happy, productive, and fun-filled life.

Mike and I shared tragedy as well. Like anyone, if you live long enough, there will be loss. Ours was significant and devastating. It was shortly after this profound and life-shattering event that Mike first suffered anxiety, panic, and, most likely, a silent heart attack. We didn't know it then, but we had stood at the event horizon overlooking the precipice of a black hole called Dementialand. And once you tumble in, there is indeed no escape. We were on the verge of sliding into the first of its four parks I call FrontierWorld.

I had been learning and changing alongside Mike as we navigated this strange, new land. If you have also found yourself on this journey, buckle up and keep your arms tucked inside the slide. You are about to experience an altogether different kind of Mr. Toad's Wild Ride—unsteady as a wagon on cobblestone, swirling as dangerously as a killer cyclone, and veering as erratically as a monster roller coaster.

Looking back, we didn't know it, but we were already there. We must have been having dinner in FrontierWorld the very day Mike had shared that he could not remember the information he was trying to learn for work. It seemed like such an innocent confession—one common to the stresses of a new job. A normal dysfunction. Chances are he had been on his way to FrontierWorld months earlier, but this was the first time I could pinpoint any issue with his memory, even with the clarity of hindsight.

At sixty-one, his energy, charisma, and intelligence were as vibrant as ever. A few months before, a good friend had hired him as the chief operating officer (COO) for a start-up company called Novellus Research, which conducted clinical drug trials in hospital settings.

Steve Kenney and Mike had been sales directors at IVAC Corporation, an Eli Lilly company, years before, so Steve, who'd been hired as CEO of Novellus, knew Mike and his competencies well. He told me Mike's leadership capabilities and strategic thought process had always impressed him. Eager to take on this next challenge—just as he had countless others before—Mike was excited about the new job and new company.

Despite Mike's years of experience in medical sales and operations, running clinical trials in the pharmaceutical industry was uncharted territory. He needed to learn a great deal of data on pharmaceuticals and the specific FDA protocol requirements for drug trials. This should have been easy for him. Mike had worked for six or seven medical companies over the years, each offering different products and services he had to learn. He'd tackled each new challenge with the aggressiveness of a seasoned lineman and the finesse and strategy of a star quarterback.

We lived in Orange County, California, in early December 2008, where we had lived for the past twenty years. Mike and I met for dinner at one of our favorite haunts, an Italian restaurant in our neighborhood. We were both tired from a long day at work and a vicious commute in LA traffic. And it had been an extraordinarily brutal year for us personally. Christmas was a few weeks away, but there would be little joy this season. The only real bright spots were that we were lucky enough to be with our three beautiful grandsons, and Mike had begun his exciting, new job at Novellus Research in April. We hoped the coming year would be significantly better than the last. It was hard to imagine that it could get any worse.

Two months earlier, just months into his new job, Mike's coworkers had taken him to the emergency room on two occasions, fearing he was having a heart attack. These episodes followed a horrific family tragedy that had sucker-punched us both. Although years later, tests would reveal there was, in fact, evidence of a silent heart attack, the doctors in the emergency rooms at the time diagnosed Mike with anxiety and panic attacks. He went back to work and, as far as I knew, was tackling the new job with vigor and determination.

Setting his glass down, Mike gazed at me across the table and said quietly, "I can't remember the information." He looked puzzled and defeated. "I'm having trouble learning about pharmaceutical trials."

"It's been an incredibly stressful year, Michael," I said. "You're starting a new job. You're just tired and working too hard at it. You'll get it, honey," I said encouragingly, pointing the tines of my fork at him for emphasis. "It's just new. Look at all the different products and services you've sold in your lifetime and trained others to sell. It's just another product training. Keep studying. You'll get it. Don't worry." But he was worried, and I was the one who didn't get it.

Two weeks later, we sat in the same restaurant. Christmas was a week away. Midway through his plate of pasta, Mike put down his fork and stared across the table at me. "Steve let me go today," he said.

"Let you go? Let you go where?" I stared back, not comprehending. "He fired me."

"What?" I sat back, stunned. Never—ever—had Mike come close to being fired. He was the star, always recruited away from his current companies by competitors. Why would Steve, one of his best friends who knew his past accomplishments and capabilities, fire him? And right before Christmas? It didn't make any sense.

Like a jet's tailhook catching the steel wires on an aircraft carrier, our life, as we knew it, came to a screeching halt. Not because Mike had lost his job, although that would have severe economic and lifestyle repercussions, but because of why he lost his job. I didn't know the answer to that question yet. If Mike had suspicions or worries, he wasn't ready to admit it to me.

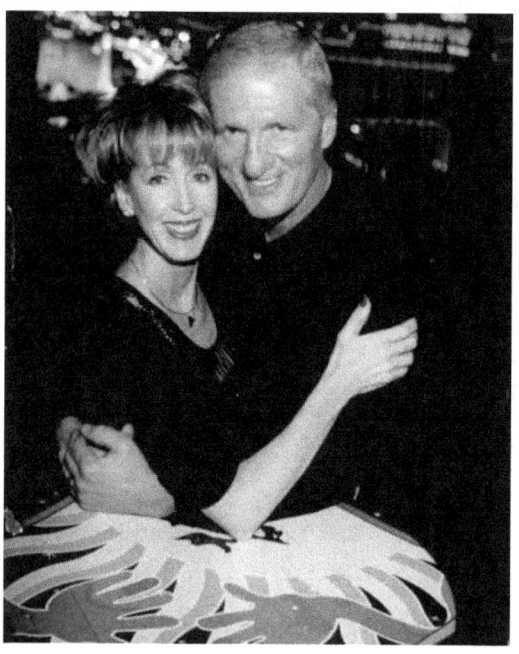

Mike and me. Happy together

Scene 2

Disneyland: My First Adventure Park Experience

I was eight years old. The night before I walked through the gates of Disneyland, my sleep was restless, filled with dreams of this new adventure park. It was 1955, but I remember it as if it were last week. My imagination and anticipation kept me awake most of the night. The tagline for Disneyland is The Happiest Place on Earth, and I was indeed happy.

My family and I stood excitedly at the entrance the year it had opened, feeling the same awe and magic the first astronauts on the moon might have experienced looking back at Earth. My parents, maternal grandparents, four-year-old sister, Cathe, and I were embarking on this great adventure together. We felt as though we had indeed left Earth and arrived at a distant star, a place that seemed to exist in another dimension.

Cathe and I had seen nothing like this in our brief lives. Very few people had, of course. Disneyland had only been open for a few months. An air of enchantment pervaded the grounds, offering adults and children refuge from their worries, allowing them to lose themselves in fantasy and imagination. Everything seemed to be awash in color. It felt like stepping into Oz.

Several years later, designers erected a copper statue of Walt Disney and Mickey Mouse holding hands. It is called "Partners," and it's the first thing you see upon entering the gates of many Disney parks. After passing under a tunnel, a big sign proclaimed:

HERE YOU
LEAVE TODAY
AND ENTER THE WORLD
OF YESTERDAY,
TOMORROW, AND FANTASY

We had started our journey by walking along Main Street, eager to enter the first land. Walt Disney hadn't packed Disneyland with rides back then—there were only twelve in the entire park. Instead, the lands featured wide-open spaces that let you imagine yourself living in the Old West, traveling down the Nile River in a riverboat, visiting a fairy tale, or living far into the distant future. Stimulating the brain through imagination was Walt Disney's goal.

Four parks, arranged in a semicircle, beckoned us to choose. Instead of joining the rush toward Fantasyland, we leisurely explored Main Street and walked around the Plaza. Frontierland, where we had begun our journey, paid tribute to the pioneers of the past and the spirit of the Old West.

As we traveled the park aboard a stagecoach pulled by beautiful horses, we imagined living like early settlers. Fascinated, yet a little wary, we gaped as the masked, gun-toting robbers demanded our driver surrender his bag of gold. Dusty and parched, we burst through the swinging doors at the Golden Horseshoe Saloon, bellied up to the kid-friendly bar, and ordered sarsaparillas and root beers to quench our powerful thirst. We watched, transfixed, as saloon girls and cowpokes sang and danced on stage in the live revue. This was indeed a world away—a world of imagination.

Leaving Frontierland, we next ambled over to Adventureland, a combination of Asian–African jungle experiences. This was my favorite park. The sounds of wild birds and monkeys were everywhere, capturing the feel of an exotic jungle adventure. This park's highlight was the Jungle

River Cruise, a thrilling adventure that twisted through the world's bushes and rainforests.

Our brave guide displayed staggering skill, steering the boat around jagged rocks with one hand while waving his pistol with the other. Dodging crocodiles and water buffalo and warning us to duck down, he had fired his realistic-looking gun at every manner of threat, including headhunters, dangerous snakes, and waterfalls.

It was both thrilling and evocative, reminding me of our nightly bedtime stories when our father had regaled us with tales of Tarzan and we read from Rudyard Kipling's Just So stories and other adventure books. Plus, Dad had pointed out that in just a few weeks, we would board a ship to our new home in South Vietnam, which had real, live jungles. My father, Colonel H. G. McNeese, was soon to assume the position of Air Attaché of Indochina, and we would live this real-life adventure for the next two years.

Reluctantly, we left Adventureland and entered Fantasyland. Designed for young children, it included spinning teacups on the Mad Tea Party ride from Alice in Wonderland. Boarding a car on a track in the elevated Mr. Toad's Wild Ride, we were jerked in and out of colorful, fanciful settings. I liked this ride but didn't want to admit it at eight, as I felt this park was too babyish. I was ready to see the future, so we headed to the last park.

Tomorrowland was where you could imagine the world many years into the future. It featured a House of the Future with Jetson-like appliances and marvels we could only have dreamed of in 1955, such as microwaves and a flat-screen TV. This journey into the unknown captured my imagination just as Star Trek would years later. What would my future be?

I have since visited some of Disney's other parks and have been back to Disneyland in Anaheim countless times. Tomorrowland has undergone the most changes of the four parks nearly seventy years since its inception, continually evolving and reinventing itself. I suppose it must be in constant upheaval because today is yesterday's future and tomorrow's yesterday.

Little did I know it then, but this adventure into the exciting world of imagination would be a milestone in my life's pursuit of fun, adventure, and meaningful love. And it would not be the only adventure park in my future. Dementialand awaited fifty years into the future.

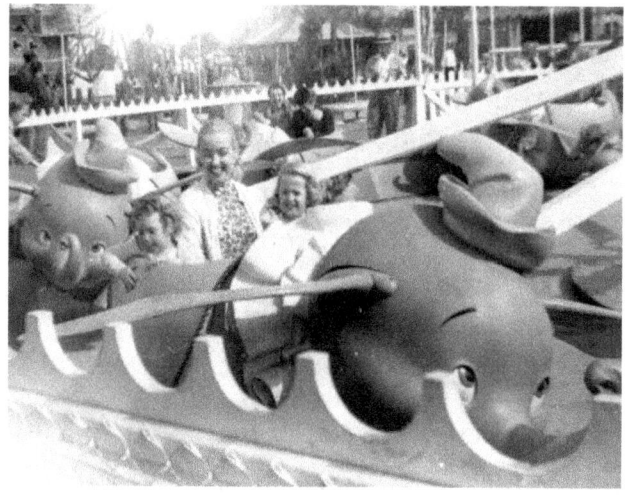

Mom, Cathe and me riding Dumbo. Circa 1955

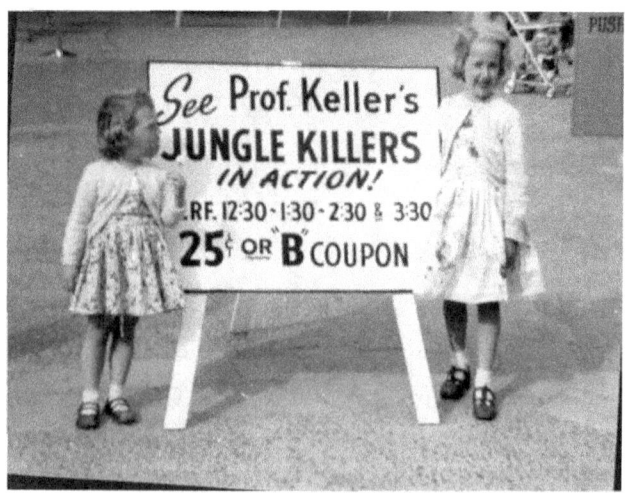

Back when Disneyland had ride tickets

Scene 3

Dementialand: My Last Adventure Park Experience

I have adored Michael Hobbs from the first moment I passed him in the hallway on the way to History 202 when we were nineteen years old and sophomores in college. He had certainly stood out—tall, handsome, and tanned. He was shy, with a big smile that flashed whenever he saw me. I felt then an electricity of excitement whenever I looked at him, which has continued to course through my nervous system for fifty-five years and counting. We have shared a lifetime of adventures and discovery, experiencing sadness, loss, joy, and contentment. Two souls forged into one.

Incredibly, out of the blue, when we were in our early sixties, Mike and I found ourselves at the entrance of an unexpected adventure park, holding hands like Micky and Walt—partners. We had no idea we were about to enter Dementialand, fifty-four years after I had visited Disneyland for the first time, and forty-four years after we'd met. This park was indeed a jarring reality that had transformed our lives but also validated our love. And yes, even in this park, we were still having fun.

Reluctantly, and certainly not by our own volition, we left Normaland and have officially lived in Dementialand for over seven years. We are naturalized citizens in an unnatural place. There is no exit from this park for people with dementia. Death is the only way out. Like a black hole—a massive, compact place so dense that its gravity prevents anything from escaping—even light-Dementialand traps people. The big, metal door slams shut, locking in the person affected. No one knows where the demons keep the brass key to unlock the door. It is out there somewhere, but no one has found it yet.

At the entrance of Dementialand, you won't find a cute, little Mickey Mouse statue holding anyone's hand. I imagine instead that there is a statue of his cousin, a big, ugly, marble Ratt, gazing fondly and with great anticipation at the brain that it is about to rip to shreds. His lips are curled, and drool leaks from the side of his mouth and down his hairy chin.

Instead of staring up at the Disneyland fairy castle that promises only joy and excitement, we stood at the brink of a precipice and stared down into a dark and bottomless pit—a Ratt hole. The slogan here could be:

HERE YOU
LEAVE YESTERDAY
AND ENTER THE WORLD
OF FANTASY,
TODAY AND TOMORROW

Though we are together, Mike and I experience Dementialand differently. I find myself straddling the two worlds—this strange, new place alongside him, and Normaland, where I and others live and will eventually return full time. Sadly, Mike has moved permanently from Normaland to Dementialand and will never emerge. Invisible demons have trapped him, holding him tightly so Ratt can dig his teeth into the soft tissue of his brain, chomping neurons as he burrows deeper and deeper.

I think of the three stages of dementia as three of the parks in Disneyland: FrontierWorld is mild dementia, AdventureWorld is middle dementia, and FantasyWorld, the last park for the directly affected, is late-stage dementia. The fourth park, TomorrowWorld, is only for the loved ones left behind.

You don't realize you are in Dementialand when you first walk into FrontierWorld after leaving Main Street. As you approach AdventureWorld, you suspect you have left Normaland, but only a few things seem out of the ordinary. The similarity between FrontierWorld and places in Normaland is so striking, you only become aware of it when you're forced down to AdventureWorld and look back up. FrontierWorld can only be seen in retrospect.

After gaining entrance to Dementialand, you might, at some point, have the sensation of being at the top of an imaginary slide, with someone slowly pushing you down the slippery, aluminum surface until you finally reach the third and last subterranean park, FantasyWorld.

Unlike Disneyland, these parks here are not contiguous. You don't wander from one to another on the same level, nor can you choose which park to enter. You visit FrontierWorld for some period of time—everyone's experience is different—then plop down on the slide and descend to AdventureWorld for another unknown period. Then invisible claws push you farther down into FantasyWorld, where you finally arrive in what seems like the pit of hell. When you enter this third park, it is hoped that the stay there will be mercifully short as the person affected cannot care for himself, and any vestige of Normaland is erased. I imagine TomorrowWorld, the fourth and final park, as a colossal trampoline that catapults loved ones back to Normaland, leaving them to face their uncertain destiny alone.

As Shakespeare's Juliet wistfully proclaimed: *"Good night, good night! Parting is such sweet sorrow. That I shall say good night till it be morrow."*

I ask myself, "How quickly will it be morrow?" *How quickly will we progress to FantasyWorld and then me to TomorrowWorld? What will the end look like? And what will my life be like without Mike in it?* TomorrowWorld is difficult for me to imagine. It's the one park that I will visit alone. And what awaits me is unknown and promises to differ vastly from anything I'd previously experienced in Normaland. That is why, for me, it's the most frightening of all the parks.

Dementia symptoms change over time, so categorizing them helps one figure out where exactly one is and where one is probably headed. Knowing what's coming can help prepare loved ones for the social, medical, and personal needs of the one affected.[1]

The most commonly used scale or chart of the symptoms is often referred to simply as GDS, for Global Deterioration Scale, or by its more formal name, the Reisberg Scale. It is a reliable tool for watching the progression of primary degenerative dementia. Developed in 1982 by Dr. Steven Roth, GDS consists of seven stages that measure global cognitive decline over time to classify individuals according to their level of impairment and assist providers and caregivers. Instead of three stages—mild, middle, and late—the GDS divides the deterioration into seven stages.

Everyone starts in Stage 1, which is zero signs of dementia. Those who are destined to have dementia will progress or, rather, regress from there. Even someone in early stages two or three does not typically exhibit enough symptoms for a dementia diagnosis. By the time a diagnosis has been made, a dementia patient is usually in Stage 4 or beyond. Therefore, Stage 4 is considered "early dementia," Stages 5 and 6 are considered "middle dementia," and Stage 7 is considered "late dementia." I have included a chart with each of the seven stages at the top of many chapters as I follow Mike's deterioration.

The path that dementia takes, and the speed at which the brain cells become damaged, depends on the type of dementia one has and the individual who has it. But it all ends up the same way. One day, the person will reach the last stage, the seventh, and the symptoms become

---

1. Dementiacarecentral.com.

so severe that they can no longer bathe, dress, eat, or go to the bathroom on their own.[2] The brain no longer controls those functions. The person is then at risk for many medical complications because they are bedridden—infections, pneumonia, and blood clots can all contribute to their death. They also have trouble swallowing, eating, and drinking, which, of course, leads to weight loss, dehydration, and malnutrition, putting them farther at risk for infection.[3] It is a horrible way to end a life, as much for the loved ones as for the person with dementia.

With the benefit of hindsight, I see that the start of our journey—Stage 2—was seventeen years ago. Of course, it wasn't apparent to either of us then that we were in Dementialand. Everything seemed normal. But we had, in fact, wandered into FrontierWorld. I can pinpoint the day in that Italian restaurant when we walked down Main Street toward FrontierWorld. I have accompanied Mike on the slide down, and what a strange and terrifying experience it is. Dementialand could be called *The Unhappiest Place on Earth.*

Stages of Alzheimer's Disease

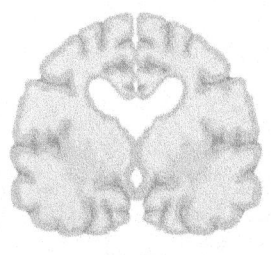 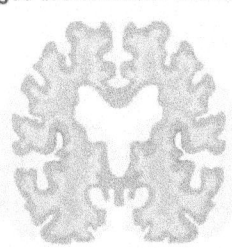 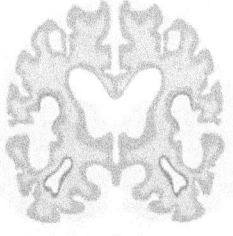

Healthy   Mild Alzheimer's   Severe Alzheimer's
Brain   Disease   Disease

Human brain MRI scan. Healthy and Alzheimer's disease brain. Healthy neuron and neuron with amyloid plaques cross section scan.

2. Verywellheath.com.

3. Verywellheath.com.

Scene 4

Backstage with the Backstories

Stage 1 - Global Deterioration Scale (GDS) / Reisberg Scale			
Diagnosis	Stage	Signs and Symptoms	Expected Duration of Stage
No Dementia	Stage 1: No Cognitive Decline	– Normal function – No memory loss – People with NO dementia are considered in Stage 1.	Hopefully forever!

Stage 1 Table: Applicable to Scenes 4 through 8

Mike and I had first collided on the highway of life in 1966 when we were sophomores in college at Butler University in Indianapolis. In a confluence of unlikely events, we were tossed together like eggs and cheese in a soufflé. The summer before my freshman year, I had arrived back in the US from France, where I'd spent my senior year in high school when my father served at NATO, headquartered just outside of Paris.

My childhood could not have been more different from Mike's. I was a bird of passage, never staying long in one spot. As the daughter of an Air Force Colonel, I was born in Los Angeles and shuffled to Tucson, Arizona, at two years old. I had then spent the next six years in suburban Falls Church, Virginia, when my father was at the Pentagon as Director of Air Training for the 20th Air Force during the Korean War. Looking back today, I realize it was an upper-middle-class, privileged existence.

In 1956, when the Air Force had assigned Dad to be the Air Attaché of Indochina, our family of four, plus our Dalmatian, Yankee, moved to

Saigon, Vietnam. There, we had lived in a French colonial mansion with seven servants, as they were called—a cook, laundress, chauffeur, upstairs and downstairs maids, and a nanny each for Cathe and me. The cook and his wife, the laundress, lived in the back servants' quarters, and the others rode bikes to work. Everyone spoke French, which served as the common language between us.

Living in Asia for two years at a young age, I had the extraordinary experience and opportunity of not only residing in a foreign land, but also traveling and exploring many countries, including the Philippines, Japan, India, Thailand, and Hong Kong. Exposure to other cultures, languages, and beliefs was an educational feast for a growing brain and curious mind. Those first ten years of my life still seem like a colossal fairy tale.

When we returned to the US, sadly for my sister and me, our parents had divorced, and the fairy tale dissolved when the wicked stepfather entered the picture. I lived for a year in Virginia with my dad when he returned to the Pentagon. I then spent junior high and high school in Southern California, where my mother and Chris, my French stepfather, had moved. As Chris tried to get a financial foothold in America, they uprooted Cathe and me, dragging us from city to city and from school to school in Orange County every single year.

But this experience, as annoying as it was, taught me to make friends quickly, and each time, I sought and connected with the "fun crowd." This was in the 1960s, and fun in Southern California was ubiquitous. There were drive-in movies, carhops on roller skates, sock hops in gyms, the songs of the Beach Boys, and, of course, the magnificent Pacific Ocean that called like a siren from the jagged rocks of the sea for teens to surf and sunbathe in its open arms, just as the rock group, The Rivieras, sang about having fun in the warm California sun.

Cathe and I moved to France just before my senior year of high school had begun. We spent the summer in Moncontour, a small French village built in the Middle Ages, and lived with our stepfather's parents in a quaint house on the main street, experiencing life in the "old country."

The month before school started, we had moved north to the outskirts of Paris to live with our father, stepmother Bara, and stepsister Cynthia. Dad was now stationed at NATO's headquarters—Supreme Headquarters Allied Powers Europe (SHAPE). There, in Paris, the opportunities for amusement and excitement for a seventeen-year-old girl were endless.

I had one adventure that became more of an incident under the Eiffel Tower while they were filming The Great Race. My girlfriend and I sneaked onto the set and donned costumes, hoping to meet Tony Curtis, the star. Spotting him on set, I raced over to him and, in my exuberance, stepped on his precious, white, buck shoes. He screamed as though I had skewered his puppy with baseball cleats, and I was unceremoniously and summarily tossed off the set.

Another misadventure led to an afternoon visit to the Paris Police Station after my girlfriend Meg shoplifted items in the Galeries Lafayette Department Store, taking a five-finger discount on just about everything she could stuff into her rather large shopping bag.

During the summer, my friend Dawnelle and I took a week-long train trip to Italy, exploring Rome, Genova, Naples, and Pompeii. Our family had vacationed in Germany, Austria, and England on holidays. Fun and adventure were high on my list of priorities, and I was living the dream.

At school, I had maintained a respectable yet unimpressive B average. I managed mediocre but high enough SAT scores to be accepted at the University of Illinois and Butler University in Indianapolis, where my mother and stepfather had recently moved. In a turbulent marriage, my mother wanted me close to home, so Butler won out.

When I landed in Indianapolis in the summer of 1965, the Midwest was new to me and felt more foreign than Asia. Having previously lived on both coasts, I had traveled through and above Indiana on my way from one side of the country to the other many times in my young life, but I never actually lived in a flyover state. I was stunned at what I considered the charming but backward IndianNOplace.

To say that Mike had a vastly different childhood would be understating the colossal chasm that stretched between his formative years and mine. In contrast, while I was frolicking in Asia, California, and Europe, Mike, born just one month before me, had grown up and stayed stuck in a tiny, rural Indiana town about an hour east of Indianapolis called Centerville. Even the name evokes an enormous yawn.

To compound the isolation, their home was far out in the country, miles away from other kids his age. His younger brother and only sibling, Ron, was seven years his junior, so the age gap had precluded a boyhood closeness or even someone to play catch with in the backyard. Their father, Roby, was a long-distance truck driver absent all week, and their mother, Evelyn, worked in a factory.

Centerville was so small that it couldn't even boast a movie theater or bowling alley. There were two bars, a grocery store, a gas station, and way too many antique shops. The boys' uncles had provided the only entertainment available to Mike and Ron. At family get-togethers, they would routinely get as drunk as pirates, swear like sailors, and then pound on each other until one or more of them had passed out.

There was literally nothing for a young lad to do for fun except amuse himself with some kind of ball. Mike told me that growing up, he'd spent hours throwing a baseball up against the garage door and catching it. School offered his only outlet, and there, he played every sport available to him. The high school had no football team, so he joined the baseball, track, and basketball teams and lettered in all three.

Fortunately, during the summers, Mike's dad occasionally took him on some of his long road trips across the country, where providence gave him his first glimpse of the world outside Centerville. With wide eyes, he had learned that there was an exciting life awaiting him beyond this dreary, little town. He saw New York and Canada through the cab window as they sped by on the interstate, then due south, crossing through Texas and into California. Mike told me he suspected, from an early age, that the stork had accidentally dropped him in Centerville on his way to California. He was sure that a better future awaited him and was ready to discover it.

To claw his way out of Centerville, he knew that college would be his only talon, and he would use it to scratch and scrape his way to a better life. Mike had studied hard in high school, making the honor roll all four years, and took the Latin and calculus classes I had avoided like a nest of vicious vipers. Outside of the classroom, sports had become his life.

By his junior year, he had reached his full height of 6'5" and weighed 185 pounds. He was athletic and excelled at every sport he tried, earning multiple athletic scholarships to colleges and universities nationwide. He was a standout basketball player who held the record in Indiana for most points scored in a half—32.

Mike had landed at Butler University on a dual basketball and baseball scholarship and almost immediately pledged the Lambda Chi Alpha Fraternity. He thrived in the fraternity's familial yet independent atmosphere. Shy initially, he felt like a minnow in an ocean full of whales where young men with wealthy parents from big cities threatened to engulf him. However, he'd quickly made friends—brothers, many of whom would stay close for our lifetime.

Free from the oppressive thumb of his overbearing and controlling mother, Mike enjoyed the social life and, during his freshman year, had slowly emerged from his quiet, rural burrow like a groundhog after a long winter.

The two of us shared some classes in our sophomore year and waved to each other as we passed in the hallway, but we had never actually met, even though I was dating his roommate. After Geoff and I had broken up, Mike dialed my phone number one evening. I was lying on my bed, reading in my attic bedroom apartment of my parents' home, when the pink Princess phone rang. I picked it up. "Hello, Sherry McNeese speaking." In my formative years, I was raised to answer the phone, "Colonel McNeese's residence, Sherry McNeese speaking," and breaking that habit was difficult.

"Hello," he said shyly. "My name is Mike Hobbs. Geoff gave me your phone number. I was wondering if you would like to go to the Cresent Girl dance with me next Friday?" He paused. I knew this was Lambda Chi's formal spring dance.

"Just a minute," I said, needing to refresh my memory as to who this Mike Hobbs was. "I'll be right back." Laying the receiver on my lacy, pink bedspread, I ran to grab my freshman yearbook and quickly located him in the photo of the basketball team. "Outstanding Freshman," it read under his name. Then I recognized him from history class. He was adorable, and his gorgeous legs were quite visible in the short basketball trunks that were then the style. "Yes, I'd love to go to the dance with you," I said in a voice that I had hoped conveyed just the right tone of interest yet stopped just short of overt eagerness.

"Great! I'll pick you up at 5:30," he said. "What's your address?" I gave it to him and warned him it was tricky to find. Two other houses were in front of our large home, set back at the end of a long, tree-lined drive.

"It's a date," I said. "See you Friday."

On Friday, dressed in a semi-formal party dress, I was still waiting at 6:00 p.m. He was late, it turned out, because he had trouble finding the house and apologized profusely when he had finally arrived. Since GPS and cell phones didn't exist, I quickly forgave him, relieved that he hadn't stood me up. How embarrassing that would have been, standing silently in the hallway of my house, surrounded by family, wearing a cocktail dress and high heels—literally all dressed up and nowhere to go. The only thing worse would have been my old childhood fear of showing up at a birthday party on the wrong day. "Oh, I'm sorry," I heard the phantom mother say in my imagination, snatching the birthday present out of my hand before closing the door in my face. "The party was yesterday."

Later, we had a great time at the Lambda Chi house and danced until about ten o'clock. Then Mike turned to me and asked, "How would you like to go to the Kentucky Derby? It's tomorrow." Not wanting the evening to end, he added, "We could leave tonight and drive to Louisville."

"Absolutely! That sounds like fun."

"Wait here," he said, dashing upstairs to change into jeans and a sweatshirt. Then we drove back to my house, where I had donned pedal pushers and a sweater, jumped in his car, and we were literally "off to the races."

Two hours later, we had arrived at the University of Louisville near Churchill Downs and joined several parties with live music and kegs of beer before collapsing in someone's apartment and getting a few hours of shut-eye.

The next day, we followed the throng of college students, bought general admission tickets to the infield, and sprawled out on blankets, surrounded by a sea of Styrofoam coolers. I had never even seen the pointy ears of a horse, and it poured rain all day, drenching everyone and everything, but the party never stopped. This would be the first of many life adventures Mike and I had shared, and we would never be apart again.

That summer, Mike went home to Centerville and worked in the neighboring town, loading caskets into trucks for delivery to mortuaries nationwide. The union boys admonished him for going too fast and told him to slow down, as he was making them look bad, and the company might expect more from them, making future labor negotiations more difficult.

I stayed home in Indianapolis, worked at a camera shop in nearby Broad Ripple, checked groceries at the local grocery store, and did promotional photo work. We continued seeing each other during the summer by frequently making the two-hour round trip between Indianapolis and

Centerville. On my first visit, his parents had invited me to stay the night in their guest room.

Mike's mother, Evelyn, was an angry, challenging woman, difficult to warm up to initially, but the job of getting her to like and eventually love me was one I took on with vigor and purpose from the first day I'd met her. Once I got to know her and learned more about how she grew up, I understood the anger that she had tried to keep bottled up.

Evelyn had been a statuesque beauty at 5'10" with auburn hair—a dazzlingly bright student who excelled in school and was an outstanding athlete. However, she had to quit high school after her junior year to go to work and help take care of her younger siblings, who needed protection from her abusive father and brother. Four years later, when WWII had ended and the soldiers and sailors came home, she married Roby, who served in the Navy as a Seabee in the Pacific. She became pregnant with Mike almost immediately. Ron was born seven years later after several miscarriages.

Evelyn's new husband, Roby, was a handsome man with an affable personality and a bit of a Southern drawl, which I am sure drew her to him. It was apparent, however, that Roby, who had quit school after the eighth grade, was no match for Evelyn intellectually. Over time, however, they seemed to have developed a rhythm in their part-time marital relationship. He was away all week driving a truck across the country, and she was at home raising two rambunctious boys and shouldering everything else. With strong German roots, she prided herself on her excellent housekeeping skills and was strict with the boys, ensuring they did their part—ironing, dusting, and vacuuming the house.

When Ron started school, Evelyn went to work. Given the limited opportunities in a small town, she toiled at assembly-line factory jobs with long hours and minimum pay. Then she went home to clean the house and discipline her boisterous boys. I sensed she was angry and resentful about the life she had felt trapped in. She frequently retreated into herself, then erupted in anger, firing off expletives that might have made her sailor husband blush. He just shook his head and smiled.

When Roby was home on weekends, he delighted in spending time with the boys, cheering them on at their games. He was the fun weekend father they revered, and Evelyn was the mean, prison-guard mom, loved but resented and feared. The house smelled constantly of smoke because both parents puffed cigarettes like factory chimneys.

Mike, I discovered, had grown up eating very little meat because his family couldn't afford it. There were lots of potatoes and fresh corn that grew in the nearby fields, but he had never tasted fresh fish. In fact, the closest thing to fish was Mrs. Paul's frozen fish sticks, breaded and fried. He'd never had artichokes, fresh asparagus, broccoli, or brussels sprouts. The only green vegetables he ever tasted were canned peas, lima beans, and green beans. He never had Chinese or Japanese food, let alone sushi. Even poached eggs were new to him. There were so many food firsts for him once he had left Centerville, and he was open and ready to experience everything the world had to offer.

Mike actually did seem like a person from an alien world in so many ways. Unlike many folks in this small, Midwestern town, he had somehow learned to speak grammatically correct English, didn't swear or smoke, and didn't have a bigoted bone in his body.

When he'd broken the house rules as a boy, Evelyn would take him to the woodshed and swat him with a switch. As he grew tall and strong in his teen years, she would discipline him the only way she knew how by taking away the one thing he enjoyed most—sports. Mike remembers many times when one coach or another would call or show up at the house to plead his case so he could go to practice, but she was intransigent.

Life is unfair, and Evelyn's lot was a testament to that sad fact. She loved her husband and sons, but I know she was angry at having to run a household and always be the disciplinarian while her husband waltzed in each weekend to have fun and cheer for the boys at their sports.

Mike had fared well in the DNA pool, drawing the best traits from both parents. He got his father's kindness and sweet nature and his mother's intellect and athletic ability. His good looks were a nice blend of each. Although angry at his mother's rigid rules, he benefited from her strict discipline and learned responsibility early.

Mike never looked back at Centerville when he had left high school, except to visit his parents. He moved into the dorm, the fraternity house, and rented rooms while at Butler. He felt as if his life had been devoid of so many opportunities for fun up to this point, he eagerly embraced the chance to spread his wings and soar like a bird freed from its iron cage. Like me, he was looking for fun, adventure, and love.

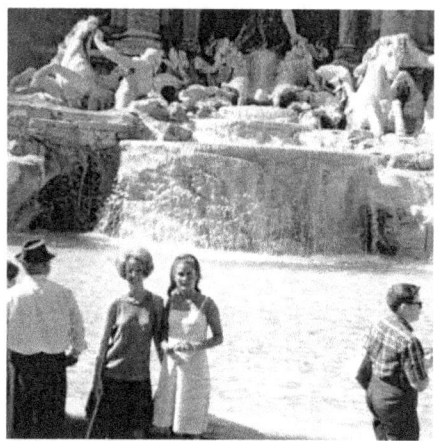

Sherry's senior year at HS in Paris included a trip to Rome

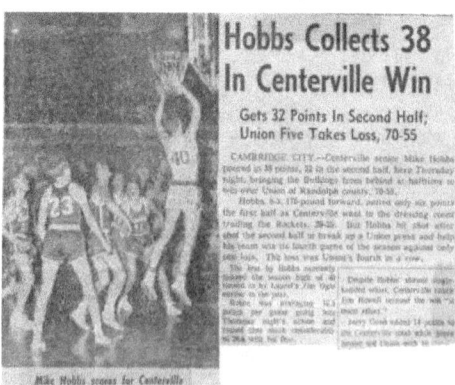

Mike's senior year at HS in Centerville included many trips to the bucket

Scene 5

Once Upon a Time

My handsome prince had captivated me initially with his tanned face, well-built physique, and gorgeous legs. With an almost perfectly shaped, lean, muscular body, he looked like the statue of Adonis that I had admired at the Louvre in Paris. And have I mentioned his gorgeous legs? Plus, he was funny, charming, and witty. He was just such fun to be with and constantly made me laugh.

Returning to Butler in the fall, we'd continued dating our junior year. This was, of course, the late 1960s, and the only birth control was the fear of sex before marriage. Not getting pregnant necessarily, but the fear of breaking one of society's ironclad rules and horrifying and disappointing parents and friends alike. "Good girls" didn't have sex before marriage. It wasn't until the end of that year that we threw caution to the wind and became intimate—both virgins experiencing our first sexual dalliance together. We were almost twenty-one years old.

Sports had always taken center stage in Mike's life, and now, with his eyes open to so many other possibilities, sports began to take a back seat as he dipped his toes into everything he felt he had been missing the first two decades of his life. As he drifted away from basketball practice due to painful shin splints that kept him benched, I had introduced him to the game of bridge and my like-minded friends who gathered in the Campus Club to while away the hours playing this challenging card game. We'd spent most of our free time and a good part of our class time in our junior year playing cards in the C-Club, as it was called. Mike had a quick mind and took to the game immediately.

As any bridge player knows, partners use verbal bidding cues, called conventions, to communicate, searching for a common suit before playing out the hands. On this memorable day, we had been at it for hours. In the last game, before tearing ourselves away for a class, Mike opened with two spades, showing a solid spade suit with 22 to 24 high card points. Without getting too far into the weeds for non-bridge players, face cards are assigned points—Aces are worth 4, Kings 3, Queens 2, and Jacks 1—so 22 to 24 high card points is a very strong hand.

Even though no money was at stake, these campus games took on a serious competitive air that drew crowds sitting on chairs surrounding the players, watching and kibitzing like old men around a garage chess game. For this session, it was standing room only.

This was a tense moment when it was my turn to bid. A hush fell over the crowd. I had 13 points and a long spade suit, which was a great fit with his hand. In fact, it was a grand-slam hand, which meant we could take all of the tricks. When the bid came back to me after several rounds, instead of raising the bid, I passed. When I laid down my cards—in my case, appropriately called the dummy hand—I revealed the 13 points and the missing King of spades. Mike gasped. "You had the King? Why didn't you go to slam?"

"I didn't know you had the other three Kings," I said.

He stared at me with an incredulous look on his face. "What did you think I had, twenty-two Jacks?" The peanut gallery erupted in laughter, and that little dig plagued me for years. That may have been our first tiff, although I also thought it was funny. It was the first time I had noticed his competitiveness in everything he did.

Like a track star outpacing a sloth, Mike quickly surpassed my bridge-playing skills with his exceptional ability to remember all the cards that had been played. I was obviously much more interested in the social aspect of the game.

During Butler's spring break, we had driven to Ft. Lauderdale and Daytona Beach. Just getting there was an adventure. We took my new, yellow, VW convertible bug because Mike was afraid that his old Chevy would break down on the long trip. Our friend and fellow bridge player, Dave Andrews, shared the driving with Mike. They were both six feet, five inches tall and folded themselves into the minuscule front seats, as neither could fit in the back. We must have looked like we were on our way to perform at the circus. All we needed were balloons and a big, red horn.

Halfway to Florida, a thunderstorm had erupted, and as torrents of rain poured down, the brand-new windshield wiper motor stopped working. The guys hooked a coat hanger up to the wipers, and whichever one was not driving stuck their hand out the window and manually moved the wipers back and forth to clear the pounding rain. Of course, everything got soaked, but we drove on, not wanting to waste a minute of precious spring break time. The rain lasted for hours, but we'd finally pulled into a VW dealership to have the wiper motor replaced.

Trying to make up for lost time, we sped through a small Southern town and got entangled in the local speed trap like flies caught in a spider's web. We had a police escort to the courthouse to pay an exorbitant fine, which ate up more precious fun hours, not to mention dollars intended for beer. We had spent the rest of the week at the beach in Daytona, and the misadventures continued. Of course, concerts, dances, and beer seemed to flow like unbroken ocean waves.

At the end of another summer, again working manual labor in Centerville, Mike had rented an apartment in Indianapolis and dropped out of Butler the first semester of his senior year, foregoing his scholarship. He'd become disillusioned with basketball practice and jokingly blamed me for monopolizing his time. In truth, he hated the coaching style of renowned coach Tony Hinkle and decided to quit the team. Even though Mike later worked out occasionally with the Indianapolis Pacers and was told many times that he could have played in the NBA, Mike was not the type of person to look back or regret a decision made. His life was ahead of him, and he was determined to be a success.

Initially, Mike had worked as a salesman for GAF Flooring, selling linoleum to flooring stores. He had a base salary, commission, and company car, and he soon became their superstar, surpassing his goals and expectations.

We married on March 28, 1970, after I'd graduated from Butler. Two years later, after completing night classes, he received his BS in business and physical education.

With a degree in sociology, I soon joined the Marion County Welfare Department in Indianapolis as a caseworker and had advanced to supervisor two years later, managing four other social workers. I then became a consultant in Child Welfare for the state of Indiana.

We were starting adulthood, excited to be on our own and climbing the ladder of success as quickly as possible. With many now-married Butler friends still living in Indianapolis, life was still a college party.

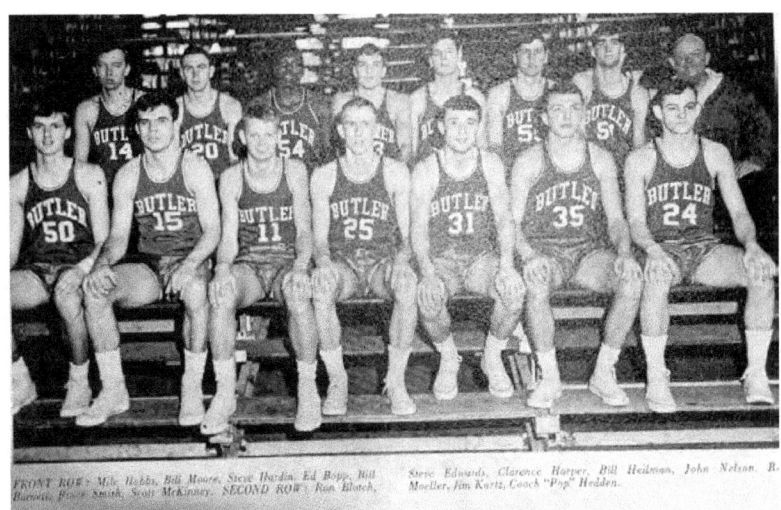

FRONT ROW: Mike Hobbs, Bob Moore, Steve Hardin, Ed Bopp, Bill Barnette, Bruce Smith, Scott McKinney. SECOND ROW: Ron Blotch, Steve Edwards, Clarence Harper, Bill Heilman, John Nelson, B. Moeller, Jim Kurtz, Coach "Pop" Hedden.

Butler University basketball team 1966. Number 50

A young Centerville native, Mike Hobbs, helped serve from behind the food bar in the press room.

Hobbs was an outstanding center for Centerville two years ago and just finished a fine season with the Butler University freshman squad.

He was a member of Butler's starting five and averaged about 10 points a game. The team finished with a 5-3 record.

The 6-4½ Butler freshman hopes to nail down a varsity slot next year.

"I'm hopeful I can make it," Hobbs said, "but I want to work with the weights and strengthen my legs."

Poised for stardom?

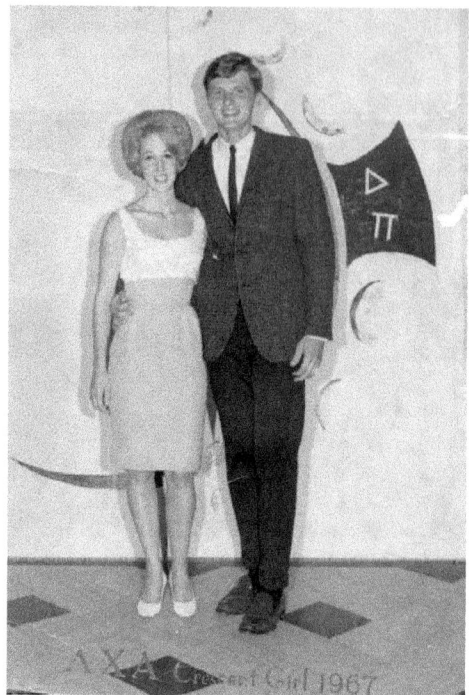

First date

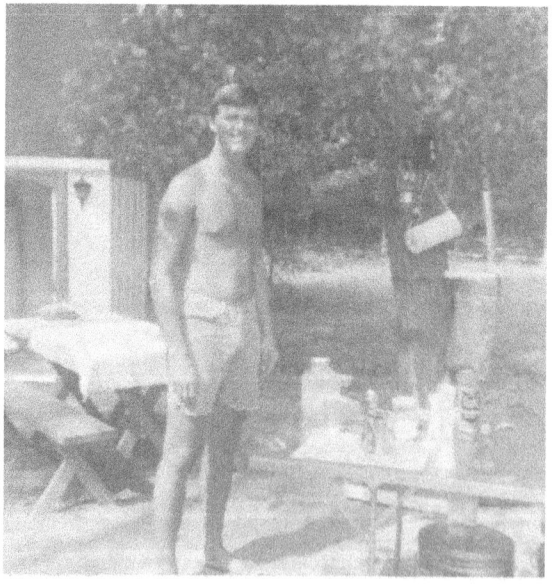

Family camping at the Kentucky River 1968

Scene 6

Our Twenties: Welcoming Brett

We had rented an apartment on the north side of Indianapolis in a complex where several newly married friends from Butler also lived. I adored Mike, and my new husband promised to love, honor, and entertain me.

Mike's handsome looks, sparkling personality, and quick intelligence made him a winner at sales, and he was setting records. Johnson & Johnson soon recruited him away from GAF, and he continued to excel, selling surgical supplies to hospitals. Given his competitive nature, when given a goal, he had surpassed it. Everyone wanted to be in his orbit. He'd qualified for the annual sales trip his first year, and the company whisked us away to Acapulco with the other top salespeople, executives, and their spouses to be wined, dined, and royally entertained. The following year was a week in Puerto Rico. Life was indeed good, and we had celebrated it continually.

The decade of our twenties was like many young couples before children entered the picture. We were busy establishing our careers, partying, playing bridge with college friends, and traveling whenever the opportunity arose. Life was just an extension of university without the nettlesome classes and studying.

After a few years, with a loan from my parents for the down payment, we had bought our first home in Noblesville, in the suburbs of Indianapolis, and started a family. I went off my birth control pills, and voilà! I was pregnant the following month and ready to become a mother. Although Mike seemed agreeable and pleased, I was unsure he was as prepared as I was. I think he still had boy brain.

When Brett popped out of me and into our lives, we were almost twenty-seven years old. Having a child, we said, would not change our lives. He or she would just fit right into our routine. Oh, the naivety of youth. Of course, our lives had changed—well, at least mine did. Brett, and my work, became my primary focus, with Mike taking second and third place. Mike continued to golf and added semi-pro softball to his weekend schedule. I was Mom.

After a while, I resented the days he had played golf on the weekends, which usually ended at the nineteenth hole, where he and his buddies enjoyed their après-golf beers. Then there were the softball tournaments. At first, I didn't mind those. While Mike played ball, Brett and I had socialized with other young mothers and their babies, picnicked, and played at the park. But soon, the seemingly endless double-elimination softball tournaments that consumed the entire weekend became as excruciating to me as hearing fingernails scrape down a chalkboard. And as Saturday approached, I wanted to scream. The weekends seemed interminable, and I secretly prayed to the softball gods for his team to lose. As Brett became a toddler, he and I stopped going to the ballpark and went to local museums or zoos on our own.

I had felt abandoned for sports, and Mike must have felt the same way. His fan club disappeared like ice cream on a hot sidewalk. This was obviously not bringing us together as a family. Emerging science tells us that a man's brain finishes maturing in his mid to late twenties. However, he doesn't reach emotional maturity until approximately age forty-three, while women reach it over a decade earlier. This ten-year gap is crucial in relationships, careers, and our overall well-being.

Among other traits, maturity allows us to understand and empathize with others, communicate effectively, and resolve conflicts amicably. [1] [2] Conflicts were always resolved amicably with us because Mike disliked arguing. He just did what he wanted. Mike was still a child in a man's body, wanting to play games and have the world revolve around him. I fumed.

Sexual tension had forged our relationship, but now, with a young son, I wanted to make sure that we grew together as a couple and as a family. I tried to find activities that Mike and I could enjoy together besides sex, bridge, and partying with friends. I treasured him and knew he loved me, but on weekends, when he wasn't playing sports, he was watching them. He loved football and wanted me to enjoy the games with him, but I could not bring myself to sit for three hours while a bunch of strangers played a game on television. Yanking out my front tooth with a monkey wrench would have been preferable.

I wanted to be up and going somewhere ... seeing, doing, learning. I had a passion for museums and art galleries. He did not. He went with me occasionally but was ready to leave after a short viewing. If given the opportunity, I could lose myself for hours in a museum, reading every placard and learning about history.

As Mike moved up the corporate ladder, he had quickly learned to adopt the social graces not instilled in him as a child. He was a good student of the trappings of success, but he also seemed to know many things instinctively. He knew what it took to fit into the role of a successful business executive.

Mike swiftly adopted proper table manners and social graces, never requiring my help sartorially. When it came to picking out clothes, he'd always done it himself. His suits were all elegantly fitted at Nordstrom's, and his carefully matched silk ties were exquisite. He took his white

---

1. Psychologytoday.com.

2. National Institute of Mental Health.

shirts—light starch, please—to the cleaners. With his impeccable taste and striking good looks, he resembled a model heading to a Gentleman's Quarterly photoshoot every day he left for work.

I enjoyed my challenging job. I had a beautiful baby boy, and I devoted myself to Mike. He had filled out his 6'5" frame, now a muscular 220 pounds, was tanned, and so very handsome, successful, and accomplished. I looked up to him, literally and figuratively. But could we gel into a family unit like carrots and marshmallows in a gelatin mold? I wondered and worried.

At work, Mike's confidence was growing off the charts. Professionally, he was the wunderkind. He had emerged from a small-town, cocooned life, exploding into a success whom everyone wanted to be around, including me. Mike was the perennial, fun-loving, Mr. Personality. I was accustomed to being my own shining asteroid, but sometimes, I felt I was just orbiting his sunny star, hoping not to collapse into myself like a black hole.

I read that stars can and do collide and merge slowly in dense regions of our galaxy. This results in the formation of a new, more massive star known as a blue straggler. These stars are hotter and brighter than others in the cluster.[3] I wanted us to merge and become a hot, brilliantly bright blue straggler. Sometimes, I felt more like a blue struggler.

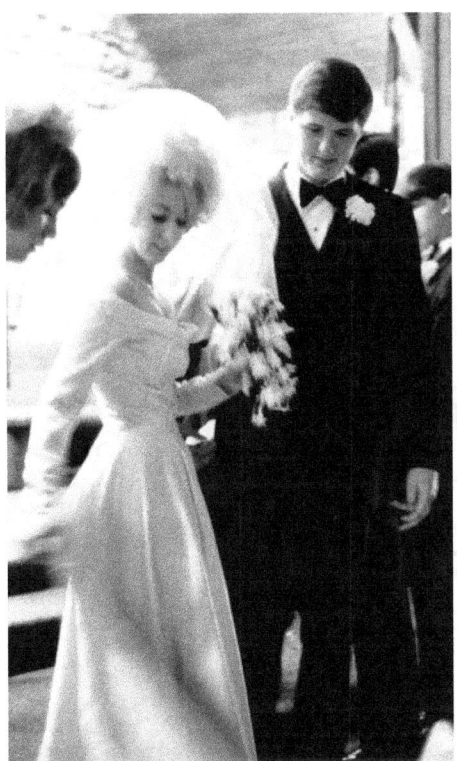

Married March 28, 1970

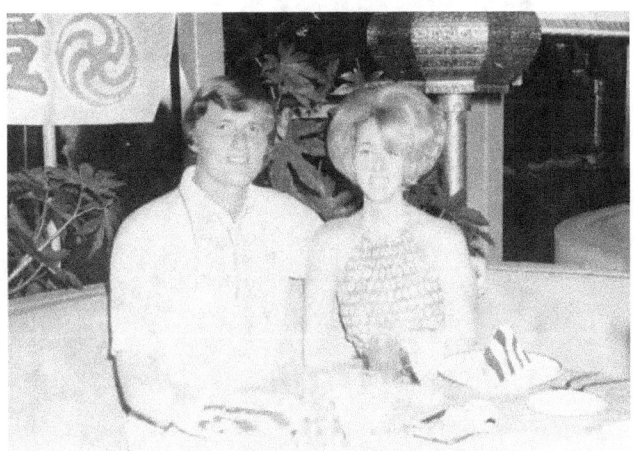

Annual Sales Winner. Acapulco, Mexico

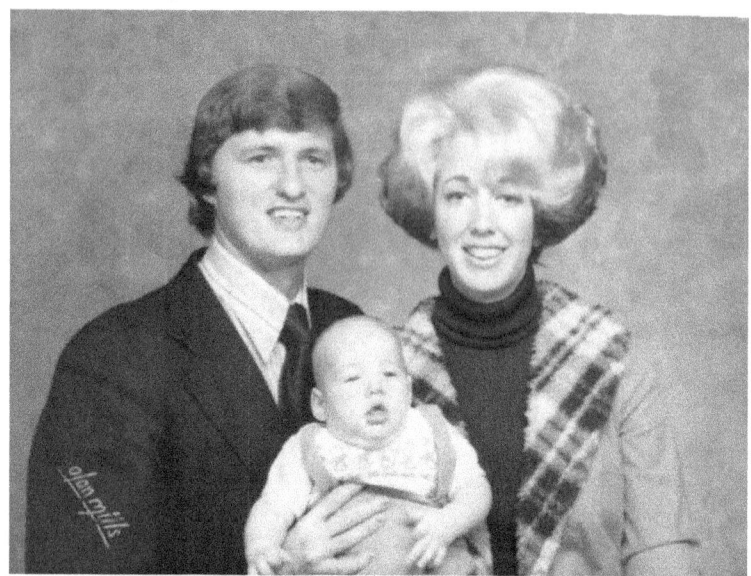

Brett is born August 23, 1974. Big hair was in.

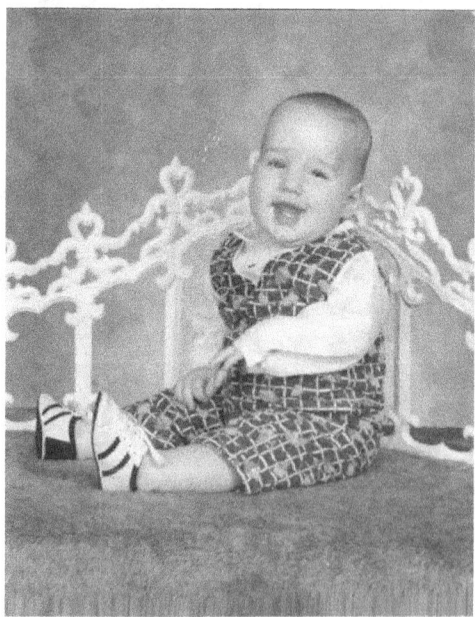

Brett at 6 months

Scene 7

Our Thirties: Onward and Upward

Brett, Mike, and I all have birthdays within a month of each other. The year Mike and I turned thirty and Brett turned three, Johnson & Johnson had promoted Mike to Regional Sales Trainer and moved us to Scottsdale, Arizona.

Accustomed to moving, I was excited to live in the desert's warmth after the cold Indiana winters and looked forward to new adventures. However, Scottsdale got a lot hotter than I expected, and I found I had to race home when grocery shopping before the ice cream melted, and a dropped egg really would fry on the sidewalk. "It's a dry heat," everyone said, and indeed, there was none of the humidity of Vietnam or the Midwest that I had previously endured. Still, if you were outside for more than a minute at 115 degrees F, it was like standing in a pizza oven, sizzling like pepperoni. Dry or not, it was hot!

The summer before we moved, I had applied for and was selected to be the director of Maricopa County's new and pretentiously named Social Problem-Solving Unit. The formidable title aside, the job entailed leading a team of caseworkers to help the impoverished, or as one might say today, the cash insecure, gain access to county services.

On the first trip to Scottsdale to buy a house, we'd stayed in a hotel and sternly warned Brett about going near the cacti. Of course, being contrary and three years old, the first thing he did was race outside and fling himself onto a giant barrel cactus. Removing the tiny needles with tweezers took hours, including a trip to the emergency room. However, Brett was a quick learner with a good memory and never had to be told to avoid the cacti again.

The home we had bought was a new, sprawling, three-bedroom, single-story abode in a recent development. Like us, all the neighbors were young professionals. With some, we experienced a memorable two-year fling. With others, we had become friends for life. Overall, it seemed like a two-year block party.

Without the softball team we'd left behind in Noblesville, Mike spent much more time with his family. He still played golf and watched football, but we frequently trekked to the Phoenix Zoo and took excursions to San Diego. Baby steps, I told myself. Blue stragglers don't magically appear. They evolve over time.

We installed an in-ground swimming pool. And while it was being excavated, gunited, and plastered, Brett and I took Mom and Tot swimming lessons. I was determined that our young son would be able to swim before the first drop of water fell into the empty pit. I was a swimmer and had learned at age two in California. Having been on high school swim teams and growing up near the ocean, I was sure that Brett would be just as drawn to the water as I was, and I was right.

Trucks and cars had always fascinated Brett, so these excavators were a special treat—clawing into the ground, throwing dirt into other trucks, and hauling it away. He loved watching the digging equipment as the pool took shape almost more than the anticipated swimming fun. He sat on a little, plastic chair under the porch in the backyard and watched every minute he was awake. It was a young boy's dream. Fortunately, the resulting swimming pool with a diving board that he raced off surpassed the disappointing conclusion of this spectacular construction project, and he happily swam and dove like a porpoise all summer.

In addition, there was plenty of adult weekend fun. Liam, our next-door neighbor on the left, came to Scottsdale to manage the family's Arizona theaters and learn about the business. His father owned a large cinema chain. Brita, his wife, was a stay-at-home mom with their two kids and had a bit of a temper that flared frequently. Even then, we viewed them as eccentric. Liam had a large, visible gun cabinet, bars on all the windows, two Dobermans, and claimed to have a black belt in karate. He was a little guy with a big chip on his shoulder for some reason. He seemed paranoid to us, but maybe it was because of all the pot he smoked.

Liam and Brita loved to inhale marijuana through a water pipe. This was the late 1970s, and young, returning Vietnam vets had introduced grass—a new and quite illegal drug—to America. Mike jumped in with both feet and frequently, on Saturday nights, the three of them would raid the local 7-Eleven before every bong session and pile the coffee table high with Ho Hos and Twinkies. Then they'd fill the bong with water, heat the glass bowl, and breathe in the aromatic weed. What followed was an unrestrained assault on the sugar mountain in front of them, and it was a gluttonous sight to behold. Like a pen full of piggies snorting and devouring slop from a trough, they would laugh hysterically at the most mundane things as chocolate coated their mouths and fingers.

I preferred to watch the entertainment unfold while I sipped a glass of wine. This was because I was uncertain what effects marijuana might have on future children I might decide to have, and I didn't want any extra calories, so I abstained. I also needed to keep my eyes on Brett, although their two older children were good sitters and entertained him.

On frequent occasions, Mike and Liam would get high and go to one of his theaters to watch Star Wars, sitting in the front row. They must have seen the movie twenty-five times through a cloud of smoke with the new Dolby sound and in cinematic color, as Liam bragged.

One Saturday night, when we were there for dinner, Liam and Brita had gotten into a heated argument. She threw a plate of spaghetti at him, and I believe he retaliated with the Caesar salad. It was entertaining, but we waited until things had cooled down and went home. We were hungry, and there wasn't much left to eat, as what remained was hanging from the kitchen cabinets.

Even their yard, in this beautiful, new development, was, like them, a bit unruly. To say that there was no architectural design would be an understatement. Mike looked at it one day and, in an aside, said to me, "It looks like a bunch of tumbleweeds blew in from the desert and just rooted on their front lawn." I laughed because that was precisely what it looked like—unplanned, unkempt, and unappealing.

Once we had moved away, our two-year adventure with the Schmitts ended. As I think back, it was like watching a hysterical animated film clip that ended abruptly, and we never got to see the full-length movie. But I suppose it would have been a disaster movie and certainly would not have had a happy ending.

By contrast, the neighbors on the other side of us would become lifelong friends. They were not into smoking a bong but loved excellent wine. Bob was a physician just out of medical school, and Connie was a nurse. She was also an incredible artist and a bit of a prankster. One evening, she coaxed me into a thrift store and persuaded me to purchase some clothes that looked as though they'd come from the Roaring Twenties, with strappy heels and red, feather boas.

Bob was well respected in the medical community, but Connie apparently felt the need to take him down a notch or two. She and I had shown up wearing the outrageous outfits when we met the men for dinner at an expensive, nose-in-the-air, hoity-toity—as Mike's mom would have said—restaurant. Unaware of the hijinks that awaited them, and coming from work, the two men wore business suits. Our husbands exhibited no signs of surprise or humiliation when we walked in, as Connie had hoped. They acted as if they were expecting to be joined by two ladies of the evening.

I found it curious that the stuffy maître d', who knew Dr. and Mrs. Cutler, also pretended not to notice our strange attire, but the group of fellow physicians and their wives, whom he had seated at a large table near us, certainly did. The colorful linen napkins we put on our heads later did not, in fact, make us invisible, but the very excellent wine we'd consumed made us think we were. I believe Bob actually led the napkin caper, knowing Mike would join in.

On the weekends, Mike and I had a jam-packed entertainment schedule between our three houses. The six of us never socialized together, however. We had friends to the left of us and friends to the right of us, but the twain never met. We all had young children, and it was easy to gather them in the house de jour to play together while the adults chatted, dined, sipped wine, or inhaled the funny stuff.

Two years later, Mike's promotion to District Sales Manager with Johnson & Johnson, and our resulting relocation to Naperville, Illinois, in the suburbs of Chicago, finally derailed the Arizona party train, and we headed back to the Midwest. Mike was now tapped to lead classes in Counselor Selling Skills, along with his management duties. He loved being center stage and mentoring young salespeople.

We were now in our midthirties, and Brett was five. Naperville was also emerging as a new and growing suburb that, once again, drew in people our age, primarily young executives. On weekends, we had played bridge and bunko with the neighbors, and Mike played golf with business friends and clients. When Mike hit the links, Brett and I took advantage of everything Chicago offered. We visited the many museums, including the Field Museum of Natural History, Shedd Aquarium, and, of course, the Lincoln Park Zoo.

Mike and I had also loved taking the train downtown to experience Chicago's restaurants and entertainment haunts. He was living his dream on top of the world, experiencing life, and we both loved the city. The only downside of living in Chicago was the weather, which was beautiful for about two weeks a year. If the wind wasn't blowing ice and sleet with a 20-below-zero windchill, it felt like Guadalcanal—hot, humid, and infested with nettlesome mosquitoes and flies. But, of course, we weren't there long before the next new promotion uprooted us with yet another move and opportunity for new horizons, vast vistas, and gray matter growth.

This time, however, the new promotion was mine. With Mike's encouragement, I left social work when we'd moved to Naperville and followed him into sales. He was an excellent teacher and mentor and eagerly taught me the consultative sales process. This method was almost identical to my training as a counselor, and I jumped in with both feet.

While both of us excelled in sales, the difference between Mike and me was that Mike needed to compete with others. I competed with only myself, always trying to beat my last week's sales. Also, unlike Mike, money did not motivate me. My goal was to be the best I could be and exceed my personal sales goals. Week after week, I did.

At the risk of tooting my own horn, I had achieved such outstanding success in my first year that I led the country in sales. My company promoted me to sales manager of this national laboratory service, and my employer moved us to my old stomping grounds—Southern California.

Mike, who had no interest in living on the East Coast, knew that another promotion with Johnson & Johnson would be to their New Jersey headquarters. With that in mind, he had recently accepted a western regional sales VP position with Medline, a nationwide medical products distribution company. His territory was the western United States, and California was where he had dreamed of someday living. My promotion suited him just fine, and once again, we were on the move. I was happy to be back home in California, if I could call anywhere home. We selected the city of Anaheim Hills in Orange County to buy our next house.

Mike had begun taking center stage in planning and leading annual sales meetings. This once shy boy from Centerville, Indiana, who started college feeling like a fish out of water, was now on stage presenting, leading, and motivating hundreds of salespeople. He was in his element, creating

PowerPoint presentations and reveling in showmanship and the attention he received. This was also the first time he deigned to have his hearing tested and finally got hearing aids. He needed to be able to hear questions from large audiences. Was it a vanity issue, or did he feel he was managing fine up to this point? I have no idea. Until then, I didn't even know he had a hearing problem, so good was he at lipreading. No wonder he didn't engage in many arguments with me, I thought later. He could easily tune me out.

On weekends, Mike had joined basketball leagues near us to get a good workout and compete with other athletes. To him, life was a series of competitions. He played at the local YMCA and Jewish Community Centers wherever we lived, pitting himself against much younger athletes. Now in our midthirties and having been married for a decade, we continued to work and play hard.

I had always been a gym member and weight-trained, and I swam for fun and exercise. In Arizona, I'd begun jogging five miles daily whenever I could fit it in. We also bought a home gym where I worked out. While it was important for both of us to stay in good physical shape and look our best, we differed in our methods. Again, Mike needed the competition to work out. I wanted to be at my best and preferred working out alone—two paths to the same holy grail.

With Brett starting school, we joined a country club, and I had begun playing golf occasionally on the weekends. Then Mike discovered the Aloha of Hawaii, and we vacationed in Maui twice a year, golfing and dining at the most beautiful restaurants the island offered. We took trips up the California coast to wine country and south to San Diego for concerts on the water. Life was always a fun adventure with Mike, and he continued to uphold his marriage vow to love, honor, and ... entertain me.

I hadn't yet convinced him to experience Europe. He said that because of the distance, he needed two weeks to see Paris and didn't want to take that much time away from work. I suspected that he just preferred golfing in Hawaii to visiting Europe. I'm sure he had thought it would be boring, like traipsing around a museum. This was a missed opportunity because my stepfather had an apartment in Paris that he used when he was in the country but was otherwise available to us. I didn't press Mike on it, though, and it had slipped through our fingers when Chris sold it several years later, just before Mike and I flew to Paris for his first trip to the City of Lights.

One evening, after a trying day at work and a long commute home, I was attempting to help Brett with his spelling while making dinner. He was in the first grade, and although extremely bright, he had struggled with reading and spelling simple words.

"We just went over that word three times, Brett. You're not trying," I said in an exasperated, slightly too loud voice.

Bursting into tears, he moaned, "You don't know how hard I try. I stand up in class and read the word, and everyone laughs at me." He folded his arms on the table, resting his head on them, and cried. He frequently reversed letters and numbers, and I had been suspecting, for some time, that he had dyslexia, but his teachers told me reversing letters was common at that age and that he would most likely outgrow it.

"It's not your fault. We'll go to the doctor and get help if there is a problem." I hugged him tightly and made an appointment the following day with an internist who specialized in learning disabilities. After physical and written tests, the doctor pronounced Brett "a pure dyslexic," which he said meant he had no coordination issues. He just didn't recognize words the way most people do. We put him in special remedial classes at his school, and he showed slow but steady improvement.

As I helped Brett with reading and math for the next few years, Mike took a genuine interest in his son's athletics. He became the coach of his baseball team and later his basketball team. We cheered during his soccer games. But Brett embraced none of the team sports we tried to interest him in. This disappointed Mike, but he never let it show to Brett. He had become a wonderful and attentive father. Instead, we encouraged and supported Brett in activities that he preferred, like building intricate model cars, skateboarding, and motocross.

Brett was also very outgoing and made friends quickly. When he was nine, the parents of one of his buddies had invited him to join their family on a cruise partway through the Panama Canal and then on to Cartagena, Columbia. He was thrilled. It was a grand experience for a young boy, and I was proud of his independence and desire to see the world and experience adventure, which I had always encouraged. In Columbia, he paid ten dollars, using pocket money we had given him, fished in a bucket, and brought back a beautiful emerald—a gift to me—that I had made into a ring.

After three years of living in Anaheim Hills, we moved south to beautiful Del Mar, just north of San Diego, when IVAC, a division of Eli Lilly, had offered Mike a job as a director of sales. During the heady years of our twenties and thirties, Mike won every annual sales contest his companies had offered. With IVAC, the trip was ten days to Sydney, Australia, Tahiti, and Bora Bora.

This was the trip of a lifetime that we shared with ten other top performers, their spouses, and executives. It was a fantastic, first-class experience, as these company-paid, organized trips always are. My mother had flown out from Virginia to stay with Brett, and she and his grandmotherly tutor, Barb, attended to his every want and need while we were gone. Everyone enjoyed the Aussie holiday, including those who had remained stateside.

We delighted in the area's beautiful weather, beaches, and rich cultural institutions during our five years in San Diego. The San Diego Zoo and the museums at Balboa Park were world class and spectacular.

With the IVAC friends, it was also a great party atmosphere. Steve Kenney, Mike's close buddy and fellow sales director at IVAC, and his wife had hosted an annual event on beautiful San Diego Bay. It was a formal croquet tournament where everyone dressed in fancy period costumes from the 1900s, and the object—besides winning the tournament—was to "arrive" in some spectacular or outlandish way. That competition got more creative every year. Invitees dropped out of the sky, got dumped out of the back of a trash truck, paraded down the street in the middle of a marching band, etc. Of course, an open bar and buffet were replenished throughout the day. These were exceedingly fun times in our lives.

Now in middle school, Brett, too, seemed to thrive. He was popular and insisted on dressing in the latest surfer-style clothes. For a class project that assigned students to describe why the selected person was a "special" person, fellow students wrote that Brett was good-looking, funny, fun, wicked smart, and always looking for trouble. They had him pegged.

Still in classes for learning disabilities, he was making substantial progress in reading. Barb Merkel, whom we had first met when she was a teacher's aide in his school, was so devoted to Brett that she became almost a part of our family, tutoring him every day after school. His independent spirit, maturity, sharp intellect, and witty personality drew him to her. When she had received a small insurance settlement from a car accident she was involved in, she invited Brett to accompany her on a week's cruise to Alaska. It was a marvelous trip for our intrepid twelve-year-old, and Barb delighted in his companionship.

I pause here to say that love is not a big enough word to describe my feelings toward Mike Hobbs. I have always admired and, in some ways, almost idolized him. We have always been best friends. He was charming, funny, and as effervescent as champagne in a chiseled, human bottle, always laughing and joking, the life of every party. I rarely remember him being angry, and there is no one I would rather spend time with. I reserved time for my female friends during work hours or when we were together as couples, but I wouldn't share my Mike time with anyone else. He had matured into a wonderfully attentive husband and father. We were not quite a blue straggler yet but were getting closer to becoming one. Would our third decade together help us finally achieve this colossal star badge?

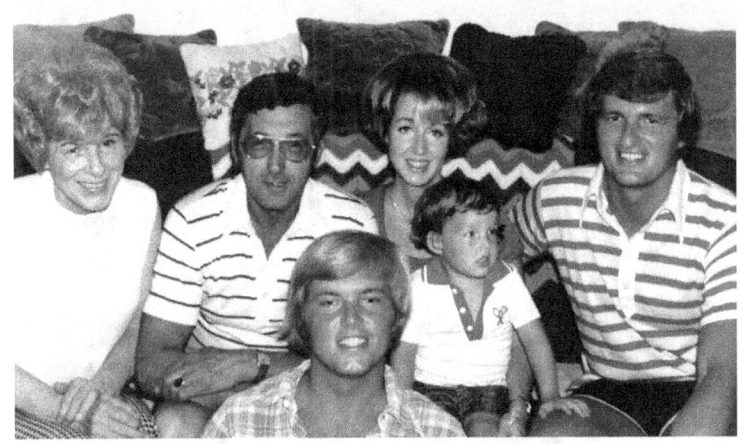

Mike's parents Evelyn, Roby and brother Ron visit in Scottsdale 1977

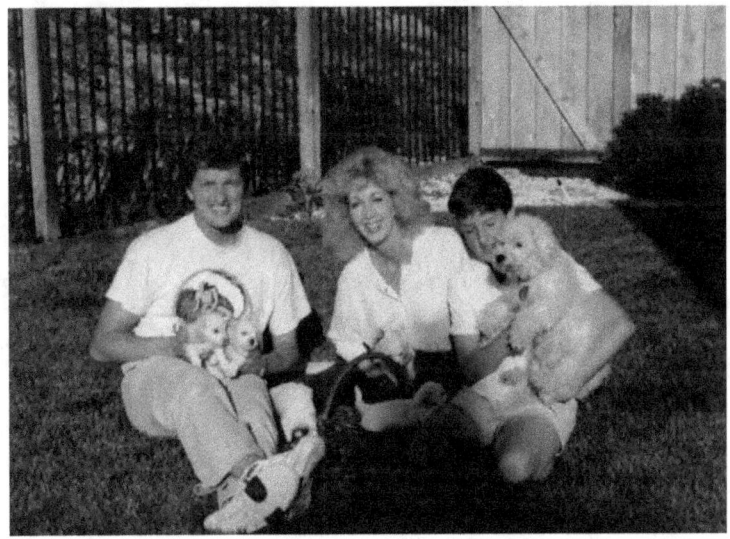

Del Mar, California. Muffin has puppies

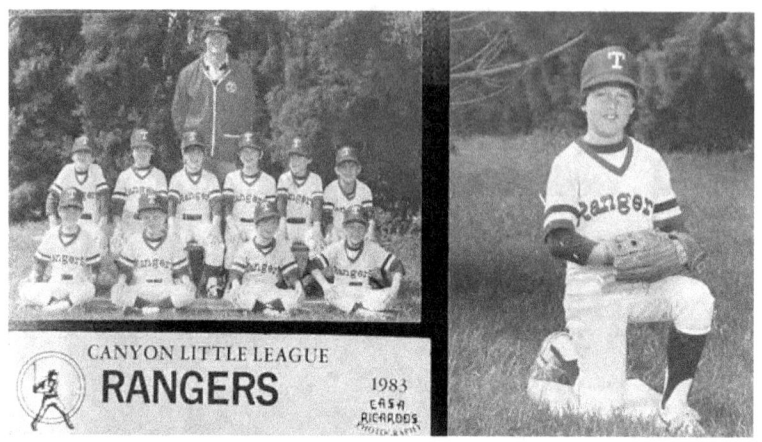

Mike is coach of Brett's Little League baseball team 1983

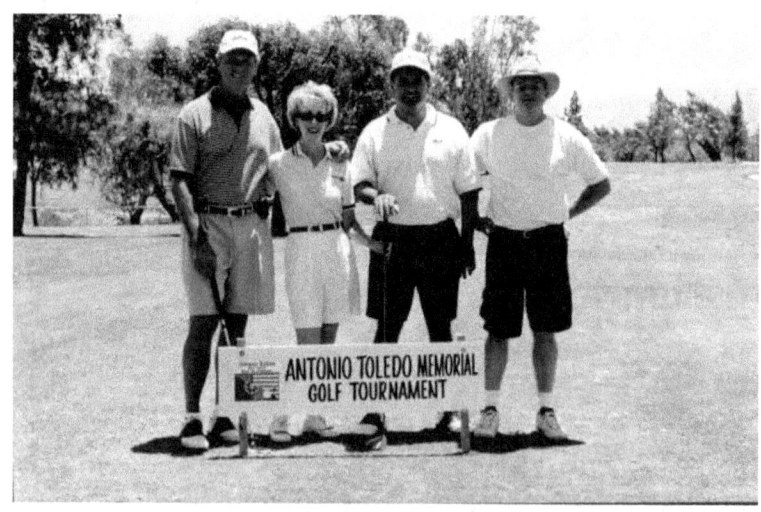

Mike and Sherry compete at golf tournament

Scene 8

Our Forties: Brett's Tumultuous Teens

I am stressed out. I can't take it anymore.
The pressure is great. I feel like I am going to pop.
"I can't take it," I said as I dropped to the floor,
Screaming, "No more. No more."
"I am stressed. It's so bad, my head is sore."
—Brett Hobbs, age 14

Mike and I had almost reached our forties and enjoyed a good life in Del Mar while pursuing challenging careers and raising a pre-teen. It sometimes felt like juggling three tennis balls and a bowling ball, but life was good and enjoyable. Of course, we had the perfect weather and were surrounded by entertainment opportunities.

In 1986, an up-and-coming start-up company, Tokos Medical, had offered Mike a VP sales position in Orange County, and we jumped at the opportunity. It was a great offer from an exciting, newly established company. Mike made the two-hour-plus round-trip commute for a year, and when Brett finished junior high school, we moved fifty miles north back to Orange County and bought a beautiful home in Laguna Hills. This opportunity with Tokos came with a generous salary, bonuses, and founder stock options with an innovative, one-of-a-kind company.

Tokos specialized in monitoring pregnant women who were at risk of delivering their babies prematurely. They did this by hooking the expectant mother up to a machine called a tocodynamometer and relaying contractions over the telephone to nurses who would monitor and prescribe tocolytics, bed rest, etc., staving off potentially life-threatening preterm births.

It was an exciting, budding industry with a young, committed leadership team, nursing staff, and sales team. Owning a piece of the company, plus having the exhilarating feeling of accomplishing something so universally laudable, was a potent combination.

The excitement of saving babies' lives swept everyone up at Tokos, and we became a closely knit pseudo-family with whom we enjoyed working and socializing. I even did freelance consulting, contacting doctors' offices by phone to keep them engaged and ordering the service. This allowed me to participate in the growing business and work from home when Brett was in junior high school so I could be there when he came home in the afternoon. There's something about the positivity and outgoing nature of salespeople and nurses that makes them great party people. It was a heady time to be involved in such an exhilarating "rocket to the stars" enterprise like Tokos.

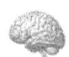

Brett was about to start high school in the fall and did not want to move. He was comfortable with his friends and classes for his learning disabilities. My biggest concern was moving away from his tutor, Barb, who had helped him throughout late elementary and junior high school and who felt like a family member. How would Brett fare without her daily scholastic mentorship? But I told myself the move would benefit us all, and he would adjust.

I had moved frequently as a child, and after all, it was the start of four years when many students would also enter the school new as several junior highs fed into Laguna Hills High School. If a move was to be made, ninth grade seemed the perfect time. Brett was intelligent, friendly, and outgoing. We didn't expect that he would have any problems adjusting. But he did. Brett's teen years were exceedingly difficult for all of us.

Without friends with whom to enter the new high school, Brett had to forge new relationships. Over time, we had learned he felt like an outcast because the school continued to assign him to "special classes" for reading and math help, and some of his peers made fun of him because of it. It didn't help that boys in the "in crowd" bullied him relentlessly because Connie, one of the most popular and adorable girls in school, attached herself to him. I learned this one day when he'd blurted out, "I don't even like her. Why are they doing this to me?" I spoke with the principal after he was involved in a fight on the school bus, but this did no good and the bullying continued.

After a challenging first year, we insisted Brett attend summer school because of two failed grades. He rebelled and ran away from home, cleverly taking the train south to San Diego to stay with his former tutor, Barb. She called, and we retrieved our wayward, recalcitrant, yet enterprising son.

Then a friend of his, who was also fourteen, was tossed out of his house. I had met his father for coffee one afternoon and tried to persuade him to come and retrieve his son, who was temporarily living with us. He was, after all, a minor. But the father had drawn a line in the sand. He told me that his son refused to quit smoking marijuana, and he wouldn't be allowed back home until he did. The man was sure his son would introduce drugs to Brett and probably already had. I was shocked and adamant that Brett was not using drugs of any kind. I was naive—and wrong.

During the summer, Mike gave Brett jobs, like clearing our huge backyard hill, and spent a lot of weekend time with him. It wasn't long, however, before Brett, with his entrepreneurial bent and business sense, figured out that he could pay Mexican workers, who'd gathered daily at the Home Depot, to do the work for him and still have a tidy profit without lifting a finger.

Mike had encouraged his interest in dirt bikes and took him to areas where he could ride. But regardless of our efforts, our son attached himself to other troubled, disaffected teens. He and his buddy Mark, who lived across the street, ran into trouble with the law when they served as lookouts, watching in the car, as two older boys stole golf clubs from a local country club. As the two juveniles, the district attorney had charged Brett and Mark with a felony, and the court sentenced them to a short stint in juvenile hall and probation. Our lawyer told us that the judicial theory was to "scare the youngsters straight." The DA handed the ringleaders, who were eighteen years old, misdemeanor charges, giving them a proverbial slap on the wrist.

Brett's court order required that he report to the probation office and take periodic drug tests, so we felt reasonably sure that he was not drinking or experimenting with drugs. Again, we were wrong. He became quite adept at skirting the rules and avoiding detection by switching urine samples.

In the fall, when Brett begged me not to make him go back to Laguna Hills High School, I assumed he felt embarrassed to return because of his juvenile record. Again, I had misjudged the situation. I learned later that it was the relentless bullying, and he didn't want to tell me. After several more attempts to sabotage the summer school plan, and protests about returning to school in September, I'd researched other school options for him. He and I toured several small private schools, but none seemed to be the right fit. His high school recommended the alternative continuation school run by the school district, and we enrolled him for the fall semester.

In September, Brett had started his sophomore year at the continuation school, where volunteers and teachers who staffed the school helped those who requested it. However, students primarily picked up assignments to be completed at home. These schools proliferate in California and may be excellent for self-disciplined and self-motivated students, but Brett was neither. He needed structure. This option allowed him to roam untethered like a yard dog looking for adventure with other similarly lost young curs. He began sneaking around with the older outcast crowd, surreptitiously experimenting with drugs and alcohol.

During the week, Mike had traveled much of the time, working and training his young salespeople throughout the country. When he was home on weekends, he spent time with Brett and tried to help guide him and encourage him to keep up with his studies. Although Brett looked up to his father, he seemed to want to be as oppositional as possible.

That first winter, friends at Tokos had invited us to a family ski weekend at Mammoth Mountain, and at age forty, Mike and I both learned to ski—really ski. Once or twice in college, he and I had tried sliding down an icy mountain in Michigan after being yanked up a hill by a rope tow with our hands dangling out of a strap. That did not seem like fun. We were freezing while wearing damp jeans and parkas.

But skiing Mammoth was an entirely different experience. We'd bought ski clothes and all the gear, excluding helmets, which weren't in vogue or in use in the 1990s. It wasn't until deadly encounters with trees felled several high-profile celebrities that headgear became ubiquitous. We took lessons and learned to carve, traverse, and, most importantly, stop. This was a new kind of sport for Mike. There was no one to compete against except the mountain, but he had tackled it with a vengeance. A natural athlete, he quickly mastered moguls and black diamond runs.

Brett wanted to snowboard, but we had insisted he first learn to ski. Like his father, he took to skiing quickly, taking jumps and skiing off the top of the mountain in no time. I was content to schuss sedately down the intermediate blue runs. I also had a healthy fear of dying that neither of them seemed to possess.

Mammoth Mountain is in the middle of California. The vast terrain—open bowls, steep chutes—boasts twenty-eight chairlifts that can access three thousand skiable acres and one hundred fifty named trails. Because it is, well, mammoth, there are relatively short lift lines, and one can make a lot of runs from 10:00 a.m. to 4:00 p.m., burning the leg muscles. From our home in Southern California, Mammoth was only a four-hour drive.

Of course, skiing is an exhilarating pastime that combines sun, snow, speed, and a bit of danger, plus the ambiance of après-ski. A piping-hot toddy warms the body, we learned. And it was an excellent sport for Brett. He could be as much of a daredevil as he wanted and satisfy his need for speed.

Soon, we were heading up to Mammoth most weekends during the long season and extended our playground to the many resorts in Utah and Colorado. Brett became an accomplished skier and snowboarder, and for several years, we'd made Christmas Eve dinner a ritual at Snowbird Lodge in Utah. While having dinner before the humongous picture window, we could watch Santa and his reindeer ski down the mountain in front of us. It was magical.

When we flew to Utah, Mike and I preferred to stay downtown in Salt Lake City because we were only a half hour in any direction from a ski destination. We loved to ski at the Deer Valley Resort, where valets were at the drop-off to take our skis and equipment and park the car. Their food buffet was a magnificent display that would shame any Las Vegas casino. I especially craved their world-famous turkey chili.

Deer Valley did not allow snowboarders, a big plus for skiers trying to avoid being wiped out by a teenage hotshot on an out-of-control board. This was another reason we had insisted Brett learn to ski before snowboarding. Options are good. The Stein Erikson Lodge was also at midmountain, where we'd enjoyed the obligatory après-ski cocktail.

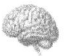

Brett had graduated from high school after taking a test proctored and coached by a sympathetic and charitable teacher, and he received his GED. But this was after he had totaled several vehicles, including a prized 911 Porsche that Mike hoped he would have forever. He had loaned Brett his car to get to his part-time job one afternoon when he was sixteen, but he drove too fast on rain-slicked streets. The Porsche hydroplaned and smashed into a light pole. Fortunately, our son was unhurt, but the car was destroyed.

We were strict but indulgent parents. When Brett was seventeen, we had bought him a black, 454 Ford pickup truck to help him "fit in." He drove fast, and the truck drew police like a rose garden attracts bees. Also, because he was still on probation, the police closely monitored him, in large part because of his reputation for speed.

Mike put Brett to work at Tokos in the stockroom that summer, and we'd tried in vain to focus him on college classes. But Brett had convinced himself he was not smart enough to learn to read well and would not be successful in college. Despite all of our efforts to bolster his confidence, he had told me repeatedly that he knew dyslexia was just a fancy word for retarded.

Mike and I played golf on weekends and had joined two gorgeous country clubs in succession. The first was Dove Canyon, a spectacular course nestled into a canyon with no surrounding homes or noises except the sounds of nature, and there were plenty of those—birds, rabbits, deer, coyotes, and the occasional snake. Then we joined Coto de Casa, which had two beautiful courses and was just minutes from our home. Mike tried to get Brett interested in golf, but Brett was too impatient to practice. He gave up after a few errant shots, angrily blaming the "stupid game."

Unlike Brett, Mike had the calm temperament and natural athleticism to be an excellent golfer. He had a handicap in the low single digits and competed for the club championship each year. He was highly competitive but scrupulously honest and would lose out annually to the man everyone knew to be an unrepentant and flagrant cheater, kicking balls out of the rough and even eschewing a sand wedge out of bunkers for his easier-to-use "hand wedge."

One year, we played in the couples' tournament, and in a nail-biting, tight finish on the 18th hole, I chunked my ball twice in the grass surrounding the green, humiliating myself and causing us to lose by a stroke. Mike related that story for many years, but in a way that showed our ability and competitiveness, not my clumsy ineptness. At least we had the dubious satisfaction of losing to the club cheater and his wife, his gifted accomplice.

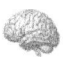

For Mike, basketball was where he was most competitive, and he loved to work out for several hours, perspiring so much that he was nicknamed Aquaman. Although most of the players in Mike's men's basketball league at the Jewish Community Center had recently graduated from university, where they played for their college teams, Mike still competed ferociously. In his forties, Mike had the ability and skill set to outshoot and outshine almost anyone.

Brett, too, was a fierce competitor. He was an accomplished motorcycle rider who had competed at the Willow Springs Motorcycle Raceway. Of course, he didn't confine his riding to the track. The Ortega Highway, one of the most dangerous roads in the US, claiming several deaths a year, primarily motorcyclists, is a treacherous, winding mountain road on which he also raced his bike most Sundays. Both Mike and Brett needed competition like they needed oxygen, but their sports differed.

Trying to gain that elusive blue straggler status, I tried to find activities Mike and I enjoyed doing together as a couple over the years. We had initially lit upon golf and bridge and added skiing to the growing list. While Mike had never convinced me to sit still for three hours and watch football games, I did introduce him to live theater. We had seen Man of La Mancha in college years ago—his first experience. Still, our careers, family, and relocations around the country all took precedence in our thirties, and we saw few productions, except for some memorable musicals in Chicago.

I will never forget the first time we had attended a small stage theater production at the Orange County Performing Arts complex. The theater sat sixty people on three sides of a compact, square stage that was level with the audience. We had front-row seats, our legs mere inches from the stage. If we had tried, we could have reached out and touched the performers.

That first play was a drama about someone wrongfully sentenced to death. The actors were incredible—we were near Hollywood, after all—with an enormous pool of talent, and Mike sat transfixed. He was so impressed that he could actually see the actors' sweat and spittle fly as they spat out the tense dialogue. The play was moving and mesmerizing. We bought season tickets on the spot afterward and had never missed a performance.

Months later, we had added the Laguna Playhouse, a slightly larger venue, and enjoyed the matinees every six weeks at both theaters. The Laguna Playhouse had the added attraction of being located in Laguna

Beach, with an array of dinner choices post-performance along the ocean. We favored one restaurant nearby that attracted the actors and allowed us to engage with them and discuss the play and the performances. We looked forward to both of these Sunday events every six weeks.

Ever the fun guy, Mike had surprised me with a trip to San Francisco for my birthday one year, blindfolding me as he led me to the plane. On another occasion, he hired a limo to pick us and five other couples up for dinner and a concert, where we'd danced with the band afterward in the bar. He loved to plan entertaining events, and I loved being spoiled and entertained. Loved? I daresay I expected to be spoiled and entertained. It was in the large print of the marriage contract.

We, and several friends, frequently took the Amtrak train, which runs along the ocean, south to San Diego. Humphrey's Half Moon Inn on Shelter Island in San Diego has an outdoor arena on the water. One day, the evening following a concert, we had entered a small lounge at a bar on the tip of the island and discovered a band practicing. No one else was in the lounge, and we sat and listened while laughing and enjoying drinks. Then we quickly realized it was Gary Puckett and the Union Gap, a heartthrob band from the late sixties to early seventies. They were there after returning from a gig in Australia, just jamming. I swooned all evening. What a treat. It was our own private concert, unexpected and surreal.

Mike Hobbs. There wasn't any adult I would rather spend time with than Mike, and he was devoted to both Brett and me. He made me feel like the star in his life. In fact, I believe we had finally achieved blue straggler status! I felt cherished, and I loved—and still love—this man. He and I were like two human grapevines that had begun life in completely different vineyards. With sun, rain, and wind, we'd grown toward each other, twinning around Brett, a magnetic stake pulling us together. As we, and our relationship, matured, Mike and I became solid life partners. We supported each other, we were best friends, and our love and concern for Brett's future united us.

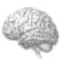

When Brett was nineteen, a local Ford dealership hired him to sell cars and trucks, which had always been his passion, if not his Achilles' heel. However, after going through sales training and working for a few months, he decided to quit the job. He told us that he didn't like the aggressive sales methods they tried to teach. He felt he was being asked to trick people into buying a vehicle. However, we later discovered that he had begun having severe anxiety and panic attacks. This, sadly, led him on his fruitless and never-ending journey of self-medication with prescription drugs and alcohol.

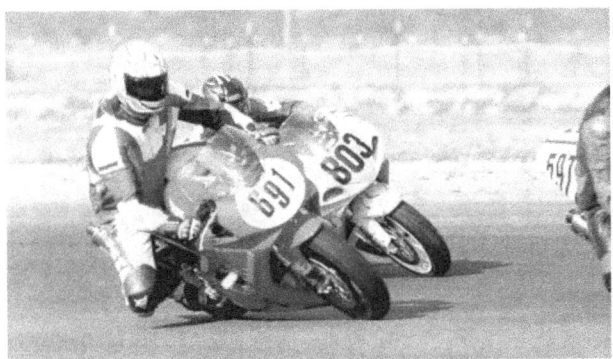

Brett number 691 at Willow Springs

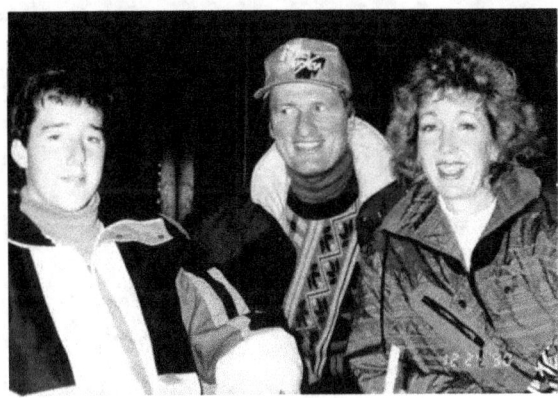

Family ski trip

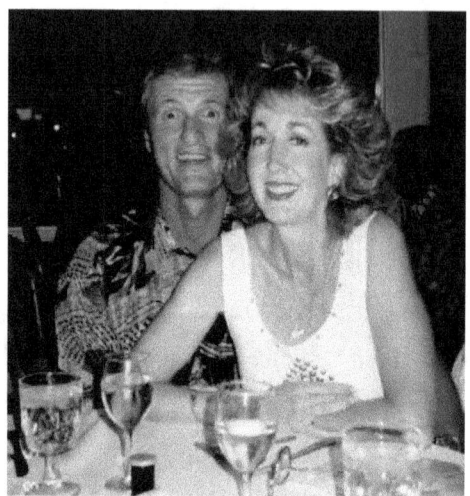

Fun in Maui

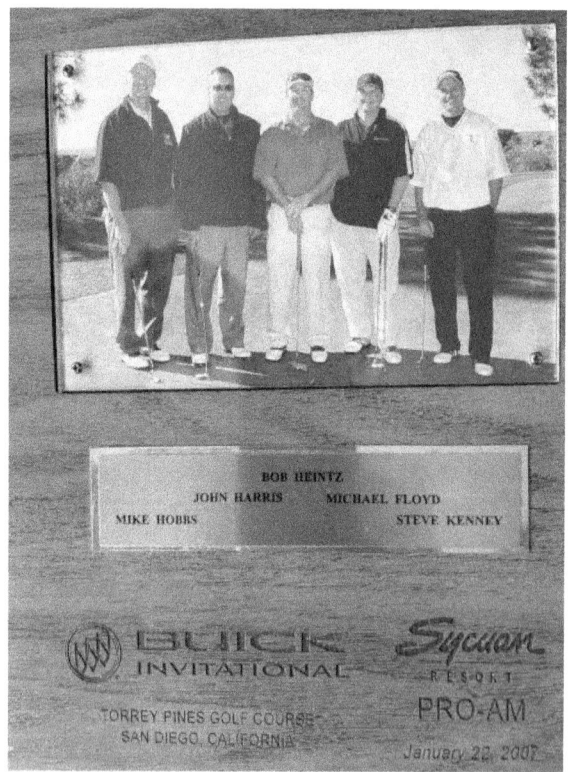

Mike and Steve in Pro-Am Invitational with Bob Heintz

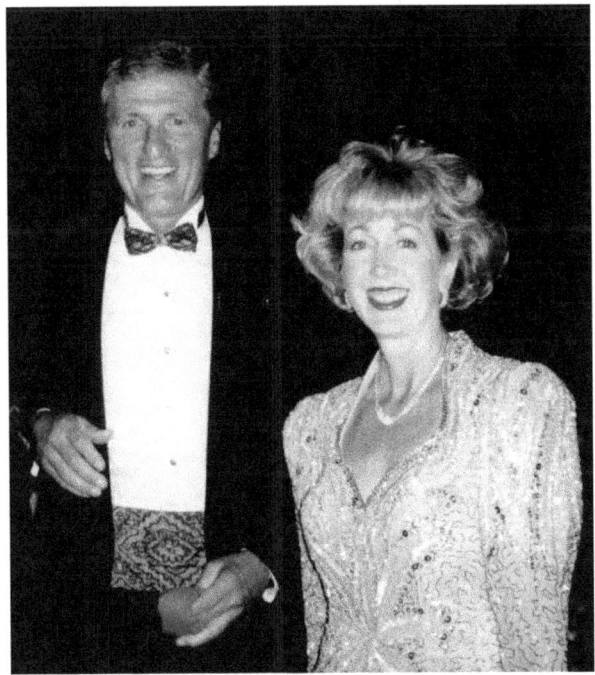

Black tie event

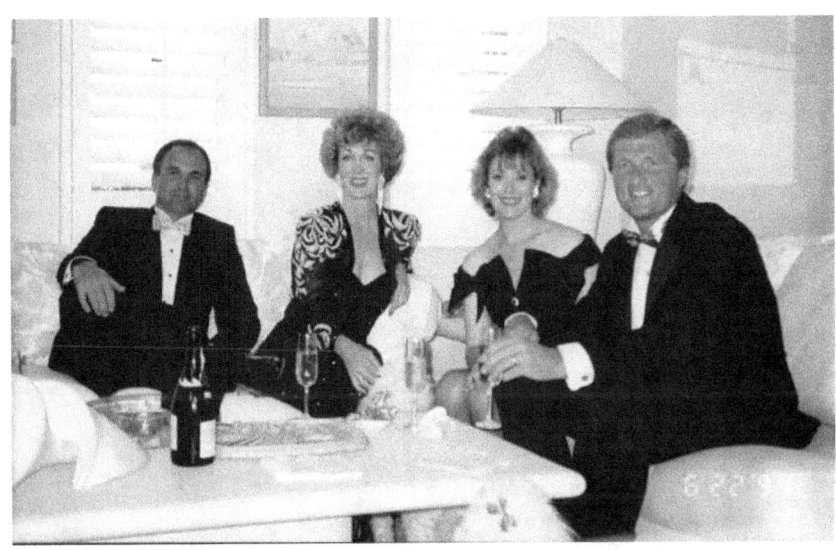

With Steve and then wife Cheri Kenney

Scene 9

Our Fifties: Brett's Turbulent Twenties

			Expected Duration of Stage
Stage 2 - Global Deterioration Scale (GDS) / Reisberg Scale			
Diagnosis	Stage	Signs and Symptoms	Expected Duration of Stage
Pre-dementia	Stage 2: Very Mild Cognitive Decline	– Forgets names – Misplaces familiar objects – Symptoms not evident to loved ones or doctors	Unknown. Very common.

Stage 2 Table: Applicable to Scenes 9 through 13

Brett's panic attacks had increased, but he didn't tell us for almost a year after he began having them. He said that he was frightened because he thought he was having a heart attack. He said he drank to calm himself. Now over eighteen, he was ineligible for our employers' medical insurance. However, after some research and a long wait, we were finally able to enroll him in a state-funded, high-risk medical insurance pool.

Despite and possibly because of appointments with psychiatrists, the diagnoses seemed to multiply like rabbits in a briar patch, from bipolar to schizophrenic to manic-depressive. It's also possible that he was doctor-shopping, too. He researched information on the internet and had become quite knowledgeable about medications, their uses, and substitutions. Since he was an adult, HIPAA laws prevented our inquiries about his diagnoses or the drugs he was being prescribed.

We worried about Brett's escalating reliance on the anxiety medication he was taking because it significantly hampered his ability to maintain focus for any length of time. *These were not street drugs,* we had told ourselves. *Doctors prescribed the drugs. He must need to take them.* And because he took them, he couldn't keep regular employment.

We had struggled with the age-old conundrum many parents face in these situations. *When does helping cross the line and become enabling? Should we continue to try to help by letting him stay at home? Is it still enabling when doctors prescribe the drugs?* Plus—and this is a big plus—we saw how hard he'd worked to find a job. His determination and drive to be successful were incredible. Finding and keeping employment, however, was very difficult for him because of his anxiety and the medications he took to purportedly alleviate the condition. We watched him struggle with the pain of failure. Unfortunately, he had also added alcohol to this dangerous mix.

Brett loved and admired his father and me and had often told us he deeply regretted not attending college and making other ill-advised choices as a teen. He didn't want to disappoint us. He wanted so desperately to be what he called "normal." We were determined to help him succeed. We saw a kind, empathetic, extraordinarily bright, young man who, despite all of our efforts and encouragements, had low self-esteem and struggled to gain his foothold in life.

Driving home one evening when he was twenty, Brett ran a red light and hit another car. The other driver suffered a broken wrist. After failing a breathalyzer test, Brett was arrested by the police and charged with a DUI by the district attorney's office. It was upgraded to a felony due to the other driver's injury. We hired an attorney, and Brett had a court hearing the following day.

Mike was out of town on business, but I had attended Brett's hearing. I watched anxiously as they brought him into the holding cage at the front of the courtroom. He was wearing the prisoner's orange jumpsuit, and I remember thinking how young he looked. When the judge imposed his sentence of a year and a half in state prison, I was stunned and blurted out, "No! Your honor, today is his twenty-first birthday."

"Well," the judge cavalierly replied, "maybe it will teach him a lesson, Mom."

And that it did, all right, but it was not what the judge was implying. It didn't reform him or open his eyes to the error of his ways. Prison had hardened him. It reinforced his resentment toward authority and taught him that on the inside, you had to align yourself with some bad people if you wanted to stay alive. Eventually, it changed who he was and who he'd become. An alcohol rehabilitation program would have been a better sentence for this young man. Unfortunately, he came up against a judge who was more interested in what he did rather than why he did it.

As I watched in disbelief, a sheriff's deputy handcuffed our son and immediately remanded him into custody. At that moment, Brett's life began to move down an irreversible track from which he would never return.

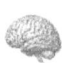

The California prison system is ruthless. Brett's introduction to the world of maximum-security prisons was stark. Prison is filled with hardened, violent men who form race-based gangs. New prisoners—particularly young ones—feel compelled to join these gangs for protection from rape and other crimes in prison. We knew it was a harsh existence for a young man with no history of violence.

"This is the real deal," Brett wrote in his first letter to us from Donovan Correctional Facility in San Diego. *"Out the window, all I can see is razor wire, an electric fence, and two gun towers. My building has two levels, with eighty cells on each level and two people in each one. In the center is a gun*

tower with gunmen. The first thing I saw was a huge sign that said, 'NO WARNING SHOTS.'"

We visited Brett, wrote encouraging, upbeat letters twice a week, and spoke by phone when we could, but it was a cruel reality that we knew he was enduring much of the time just trying to stay alive. He rarely talked about his experiences on the inside.

After almost a year in prison, Brett was released early and had difficulty finding regular employment. He had no formal education beyond his GED, a prison record, and a suspended driver's license. His brilliance and creativity were genuine, and his IQ had been tested at nearly genius level. With his dad's help writing the business plan, he'd launched several innovative internet ventures. For over a decade, he and Mike worked side by side almost every weekend. We were determined to help him succeed in life.

One business they had started was an internet salvage parts company that Brett called Salnet. Mike wrote the business plan, researched the marketing, and kept the books. He and Brett were bound by a connection as strong as any father and adult son could have.

At twenty-four, Brett was again incarcerated for a parole violation—drinking. Between stints in prison, he'd lived with us for all but a few months when he and a girlfriend rented a home. Like all of his relationships, however, this one was short-lived. He had fathered three sons with two other young women, Sunneshine and Tracy. Although he tried, his anxiety, medications, and struggles with impulsiveness and focus prevented him from lasting relationships or steady employment. The drug use in his teenage years had probably hindered his maturation process, akin to using herbicide instead of water on a developing lily.

Davin, his first son, was a year old at the time Brett went back to prison, and Sunneshine was pregnant with their second son, Corben. He and Sunne had previously agreed that Brett would have custody of Davin on the weekends, and since Brett lived with us when he wasn't jailed, we became Davin's and later Corben's devoted weekend caretakers by proxy.

This was a "job" that Mike and I took on with great pleasure. We were enraptured spending our weekends with our grandsons as babies, then toddlers, and later as engaging, delightful, young boys who were bright and eager to learn and explore the world. I wonder if, in some small way, Mike felt this was atonement for the years of weekends he had spent playing golf or baseball when Brett was young and partly blamed himself for his problems. Regardless, he devoted himself to his grandsons, eagerly looking forward to weekends with them as much as I did.

When Brett came home after this second prison sentence on a parole violation, he had muscled his 6'2" 220-pound frame into a bodybuilder's physique. At home, he continued to lift weights, studied nutrition, and took protein supplements and vitamins. He loved good art and began to cover his body with professionally inked tattoos, like a mobile montage of masterpieces. Thankfully, from our point of view, he never engraved his face, neck, or hands and assured us he wouldn't. Ever hopeful, he wanted to keep them coverable for job prospects. Mike and I were from the generation before tattoos were acceptable or ubiquitous, but we never criticized him for his body art. As he kept adding artwork, he told us tattooing was like another addiction for him.

Each time Brett returned from prison, he became harder and more resentful of authority. This time, he had shaved his head, adding to his bad boy reputation and appearance and diminishing our hopes of him integrating into a life of respectability and achievement.

The only positive outcome of these prison sentences was that he'd become an avid reader. *What a cruel irony,* I thought. He was in prison in part because he struggled to read, and now, prison was the vehicle that forced him to learn that very skill.

With nothing but time and trapped inside a small cell, Brett read whatever he could get his hands on from the prison library and then asked us to send him books weekly. His favorite authors were Hemingway, James A. Michener, and Mario Puzo. He loved James Clavell's Shōgun and its six-volume saga about ancient Japan. History fascinated him. In his bedroom at home, he assiduously watched the History Channel and listened to the BBC news to get a world perspective of events. I have often lamented what an outstanding student he could have been in college if his life had taken a different turn or if he had made different choices in his teens.

After missing an annual pap smear, I was diagnosed with non-HPV cervical cancer and, at fifty-four, underwent a total hysterectomy. I mention this because both Brett and Mike were so distraught. Brett visited me every day while I was in the hospital and took great interest in my recovery. He had many reasons to have anxiety—a prison record, no job, no prospects, three children ... The thought that his mother might die just added to his list. Fortunately, with the removal of the tumor, followed by radiation, I have been cancer-free ever since.

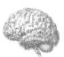

In what turned out to be a final, desperate attempt to help our son create a lasting business with which he could become self-sufficient, we had refinanced our home, bought a van with the equity, and had it specially retrofitted with all the equipment needed for carpet cleaning.

Brett and his friend Todd, who had some experience working for a carpet cleaning company, firmly believed they could build Qual-Tec Carpet Cleaning into a thriving business. Again, Mike worked tirelessly to help him by writing his business plan and securing advertisements and marketing opportunities. Brett had actually taken a six-week carpet cleaning technician course and received his certification. Considering his disdain for formal education and his inability to stay focused on anything for very long, we were almost as proud of him as we would have been if he had graduated from college *summa cum laude*. He printed beautiful business cards, which they advertised in the local, upscale county magazine, and the business seemed to take off.

The two young men began their carpet cleaning enterprise with quite a few customers, particularly our friends Paul and Linda Lapine, who kindly had their carpets cleaned by Qual-Tec at least twice a month to help Brett succeed. However, like all of his business efforts, he was ill-equipped to do the everyday tasks required to build a repeat customer base (other than the Lapines) and create a lasting service business. He became impatient with the minutia of maintaining a customer base, and ultimately, the company had failed when Brett went back to prison for his third and last stint on yet another parole violation for possession of alcohol.

Besides his father and me, Brett had many close male and female friends. While some were successful and educated, others were on the unsavory side. Brett had an incredible charm and was delightful to be around in his manic mode. He was also empathetic and cared deeply about others. He had a close female friend, Kristy, whom he was constantly counseling, trying to help her solve her life's problems. I found it endearing but, sadly, ironic—the blind leading the blind.

Whenever Brett was in prison, we had connected mainly through letter-writing, typing long, heartfelt, encouraging letters to keep him informed about the activities of his young sons. He wrote back faithfully. We visited him whenever the prisons were geographically feasible to access, but the system moved him around frequently.

When he was home, Brett had often participated in weekend activities with the boys, but as his anxiety and depression set in, he spent much of his time sleeping. I planned trips to the zoo, Legoland, San Diego, or the beach, where Brett occasionally joined us and took part as they got older. Mike and I loved those boys through a decade of delightful weekends.

For me, having these two young mounds of Play-Doh to help mold and take on adventures was a dream come true. I'd always related to Auntie Mame prodding Agnes Gooch, "Live! Life is a banquet, and most poor suckers are starving." Just as I had done with Brett, I wanted them to experience everything—museums, zoos, plays, aquariums, and the world. Every weekend was a joyous adventure with these eager disciples as we revealed the world's possibilities and broadened their perspectives. Before Corben was born, I took Sunne and Davin on a visit to Washington, DC. We stayed with my mom in Falls Church, Virginia, and toured the many sites in the nation's capital.

The boys loved playing in our backyard as toddlers, where a Jacuzzi served as a small swimming pool. We had also installed a large sandpit and playground with swings and a slide. They had their own bedroom in our home, complete with bunk beds, a toy table, and a colorful Spiderman that I painted on the wall. We read to them at night, just like my parents did with me and we had done with Brett, making sure they had plenty of books to encourage their passion for learning. We trekked to the neighborhood swimming pool down the street and hiked the great nature trails within walking distance of the house.

We would include Gavin, Brett's third son, whenever we could, but we had a more distant relationship with his mother, Tracy, and Gavin lived with her parents, who had custody of him. We were cordial, but it was a bit of an awkward situation during those early years.

All three boys loved building with Legos and were incredibly good at designing intricate structures and roadways for toy cars. I bought a gigantic bag of miscellaneous Lego parts on the internet, and as they grew, they'd spent hours designing and crafting imaginative structures and cities. Sunneshine's grandfather Lynn and uncles were architects, and Davin and Corben definitely inherited their artistic architectural construction genes.

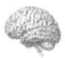

The following letter from Brett was written from prison. This was his second stint for parole violations, his third time in prison. He was twenty-nine.

September 2, 2003

   Dear Dad,

   I just wanted to let you know how much I appreciate all you have done for me and for not shooting me in the face with a bazooka. I think back on all the shitty things I put you through in my life—drugs, outrageous behavior, juvenile hall, dropping out of school, bad friends, late nights, police, cars, cars, cars, county jail, state prison, alcohol, and, most important, disrespect. That is way more than any one family—except maybe the Manson family—should have to deal with. But I will make you this promise. Everything will turn out better than you think.

   Also, I want you to know that all the great values that you and Mom have hammered into me did not go in one ear and out the other. They just lay dormant for a while. And all those values will end up where they matter most—in Davin, Corben, and Gavin, "my perfect angels." Wow! I can't wait for their teen years. And yes, I might have to borrow that bazooka since it's just lying around.

   I love you so, so much.

   The good son,

   Brett

September 10, 2003

Dear Brett,

Thank you so much for this letter! I cannot aptly express in words how much it means to me. It made me laugh, and it made me cry, like the best novels we read and the best movies we watch over and over again. I am keeping this letter in a safe place. It means that much, and I appreciate you taking the time to reach out the way you have.

Hopefully, you have always known that we never have, and never will, give up on you. Mom and I deeply regret that we could not totally understand the physical and emotional pain and confusion you were enduring over the past few years. We have always known, without question, that you have a big heart, a strong social conscience, a great personality, and a brilliant mind. Therefore, with the right help, you have a bright future. You are well on your way!

Having said that, I want you to please not be so hard on yourself! First, the past is all water over the dam. Second, as you know, you cannot change the past, so remain focused only on moving forward (as you have). You continue to demonstrate great character and resolve in times of hardship. Most people don't have that kind of emotional strength and endurance. It takes courage to acknowledge and admit your past mistakes and a strong will to do what you must to address and avoid any further distractions.

Most of us start out in life not knowing what our means of livelihood will be. No matter what direction one chooses, it is a distant second in importance to being a great parent. I am pleased and proud of your focus on moving forward with the primary focus on your boys. The other stuff will fall into place. Trust me on that one.

Mom and I have been out of town recently but will be home for the next two weeks, starting Monday, September 15th. I am planning to visit you on

Friday, and I believe Mom is planning to bring the kids that weekend. I will hold off on future news until I see you next week.

Talk to you soon. And, by the way, I got rid of the bazooka. You won't need it.

Much love,

Dad

This third time, the court had sentenced Brett to a low-level prison for drug and alcohol offenders an hour from the house, and we took Davin and Corben, ages three and five, to visit him every weekend. It was ironic, Brett told us later, that the facility for drug and alcohol offenders had more drugs readily available to the prisoners than any other prison he had been incarcerated in.

In terms of visitation, the upside was that this was not a typical prison, as visitors met with the prisoners in an open courtyard at picnic tables instead of an enclosed booth with a glass partition. The boys were always so excited to see Dad. We told them he worked for the state and couldn't come home, but we could visit him. This meant leaving the house at 4:00 a.m., driving an hour to get to the prison, and then cooling our heels for two hours in an outdoor tented area for families queuing up for visitation.

We took books and games for the boys to play with while we waited. Like farm animals being herded, we were finally ushered through metal detectors and into the visitors' area, where we spent a few hours with Brett. The boys didn't care about the long waits. They were excited to see Dad.

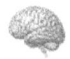

Mike and I enjoyed taking Davin and Corben on various weekend adventures. We rode the Amtrack train south to San Diego to visit the San Diego Zoo and museums in Balboa Park, and north to Los Angeles, visiting La Brea Tar Pits, where dinosaur bones bubbled up. We toured art galleries and took other exciting day trips throughout the Los Angeles area. We exposed the boys to live theater with children's productions.

When they had reached ages six and eight, we made it a Sunday ritual to ride bikes five miles into the neighboring town of Rancho Santa Margarita and enjoy breakfast or lunch before cycling back to the house. Sunday nights before Sunneshine picked them up, we traditionally drove to our favorite pizza restaurant, Sonny's, in San Clemente, and stopped for frozen yogurt afterward on the way home.

Brett drifted into his thirties, and without any work prospects, he started going out partying at night more frequently. Dressed like a prince, he put on a happy, successful face and patronized bars in Laguna and Newport Beach, where the rich and famous hung out, delighting and entertaining everyone in his orbit. And he knew everyone. During the day, however, he was increasingly depressed and slept a good deal of the time.

He was so charismatic and colorful that a young TV producer had signed him to act in a new reality show about seven single men in Newport Beach. Brett was now thirty-two, a big guy with a shaved head, a deep voice, and covered in tattoos—a more heavily tatted white version of Dwayne "The Rock" Johnson. He was handsome, funny, and knew how to charm the ladies, but he had little to offer any woman interested in a long-term relationship. My heart broke for him as he struggled to understand this reality.

For Brett, everything hinged on this reality show. He was convinced that this was the linchpin that would magically transform his life for the better. He and the other prospective cast members had attended a big launch party hosted by the producer at the Ritz Carlton in Newport Beach. Video from that event later revealed that he was the life of the party, interviewing and being interviewed—charming, witty, and inebriated.

I left work the following day when he'd called to ask me for a ride home from the Ritz. He said his car and watch had been stolen. I felt such a deep sadness for him and his life. Whenever something positive and hopeful happened to him, it was followed by some disastrous event. It was as if a storm cloud hung perpetually over his head, yet he was the warm air causing the cloud to form, and he couldn't seem to get out of his own way.

As I pulled up to the beautiful entrance of the Ritz, my son sat on a curb, holding his head in his hands. He was, of course, hungover. The watch was never recovered, and it was days before the car was discovered in a valet parking lot. He had forgotten that he didn't self-park.

Before the first episode of this reality show was filmed, Brett learned he was looking at another prison sentence of likely twelve months. When he thought about the show hiring another actor before his release in a year, he felt devastated and depressed. I tried to bolster him by suggesting they might wait or include the stay as part of the show, but he believed it would completely destroy his reputation and life. We just didn't know how deeply depressed he had become.

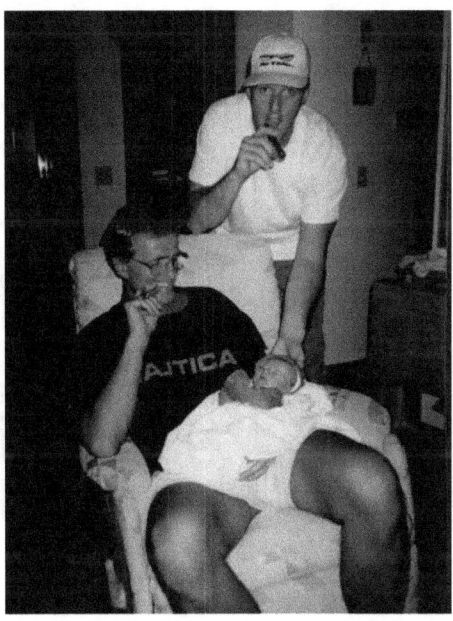

Welcoming Davin

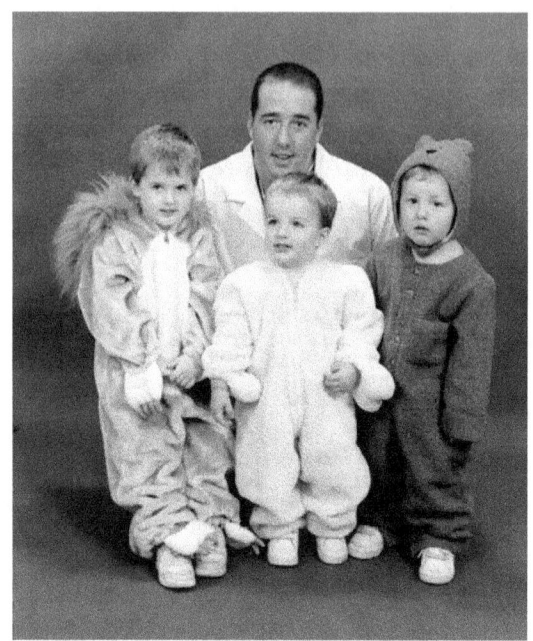

Halloween with his three babies

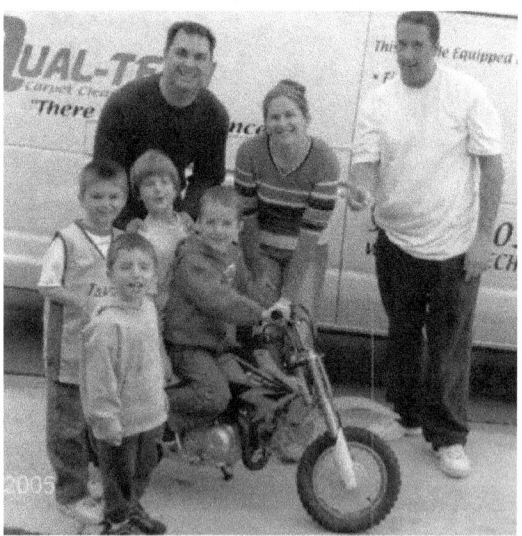

Brett with Qual-Tec carpet cleaning truck

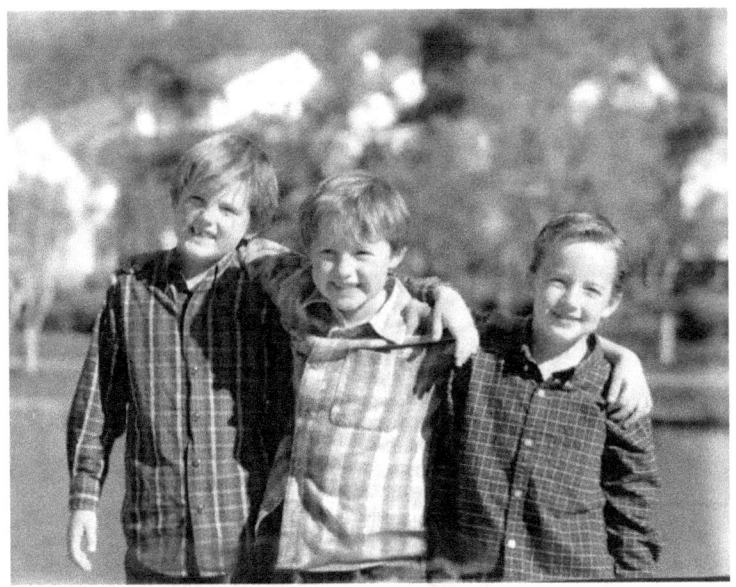

Davin, Gavin and Corben

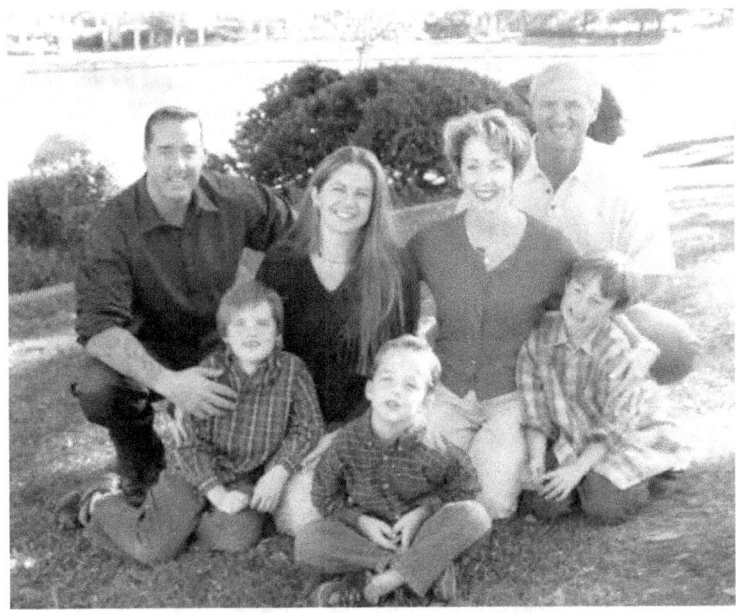

The family

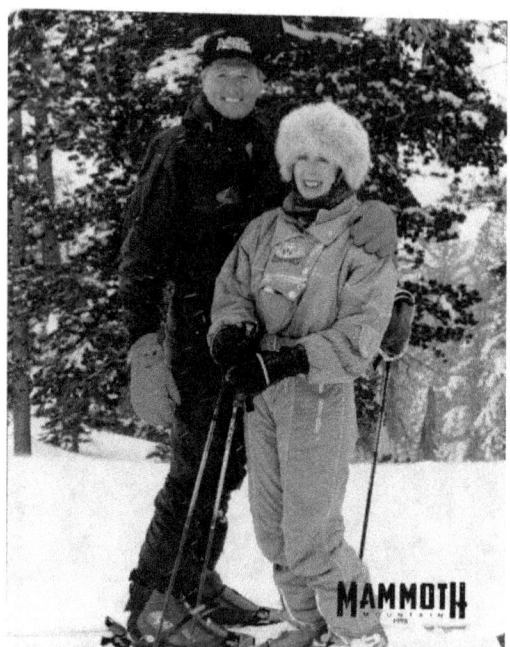

Skiing at Mammoth

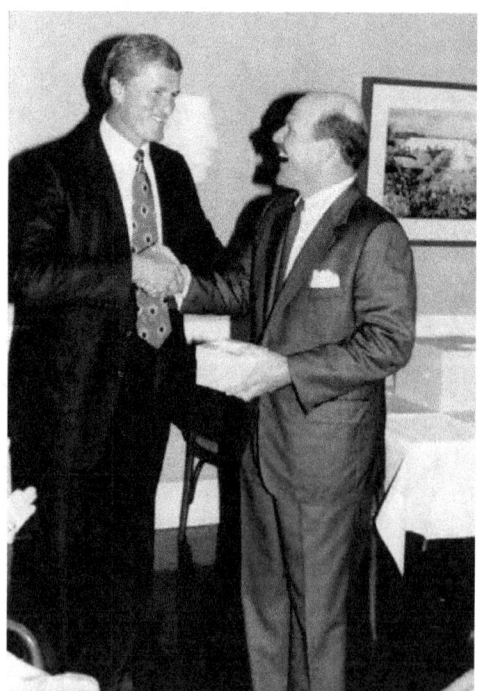

Mike receiving award from Craig Davenport, President of Tokos

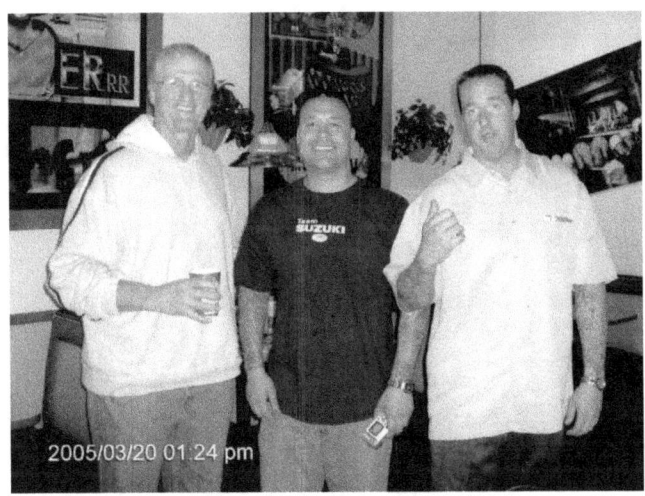

Brett, Mike and friend Eddie

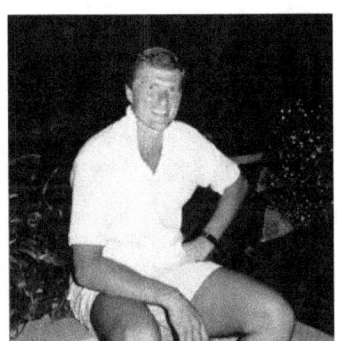

Life is good

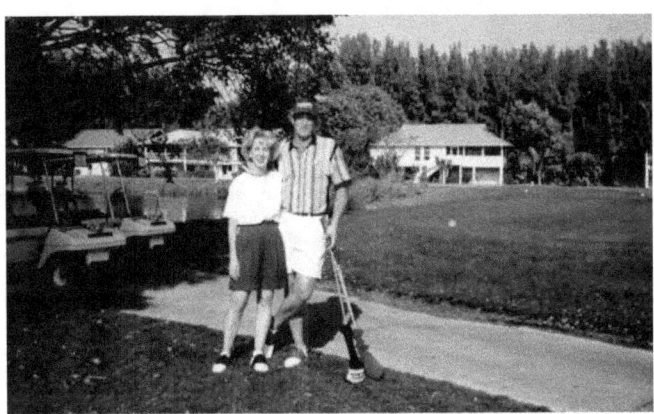

Hitting the links

Scene 10

The Life-Altering Call

After ten years, Tokos Medical was sold to another company, and we cashed out our stock options for a handsome sum. Mike and his good friend Charlie Hearn started their own medical company, Maternicare, which also focused on women's health during pregnancy. Mike wrote the business plan and secured seed money. He was president, and Charlie was vice president.

After a year, they had accepted a sizable investment offer from a venture capital company, which we later discovered was a misnomer. Vulture Capital Company was much more accurate. With majority control, they'd fired the only two people who knew anything about the business and put in their own talon-picked buzzards. Maternicare soon became carrion.

In the intervening years, Mike took executive positions in several start-up companies. These companies, which offered the initial founder's stock and had the potential to pay off big time with the right effort, team, product, or service, always intrigued Mike. He had an entrepreneurial spirit, and it was all about competition.

So, in April 2008, when longtime friend Steve Kenney, who had been chosen to be president of a new drug trial company called Novellus, was hand-picking his team, he reached out to Mike and offered him the position of COO—chief operating officer. Mike jumped at the chance and started on April 15, 2008. His responsibilities included business development, operations, and strategic planning.

The risk–reward potential with Novellus was a favorable balance. This seemed like a great opportunity. The money was good, the potential stock options lucrative, and Mike would again work with people he knew and enjoyed being around. While he had never been involved in drug trials, he and Steve had, of course, worked together at IVAC, an Eli Lilly company. And he was bright and a quick study. He just needed to learn the products and the process. He brought home reams of information and set about learning. Easy, we thought.

A month and a half after Mike had accepted the position with Novellus, we flew back to Indiana to help his father, Roby. He had been living by himself since Mike's mother, Evelyn, passed away in 2007, and he was not coping well. Due to a lifetime of smoking, he had acquired COPD and was tethered to an oxygen tank. He was also unaccustomed to living alone, missed Evelyn, and had begun to drink heavily.

Since he continued to smoke, this was a disaster waiting to happen. We, including Roby, felt assisted living would be best for him, where he would have meals prepared and his room cleaned regularly. We tried to convince him to come live with or near us, but he was stubborn as a country mule and wanted to stay in Centerville. The facility where Evelyn had spent her last year was nearby. He knew the entire staff well, and that's where he wanted to live.

We tried to convince Brett to come with us to Indiana and visit his grandfather, but he demurred. Thursday night, we called to check in on him while we were away, and he sounded upbeat. "I'm doing fine, Mom," he had said. "Todd's coming over tonight, and we're just going to have a few beers and order a pizza." Todd was a college student, home for the summer, who lived across the street with his parents. I handed the phone to Mike, and they briefly discussed Brett's latest plans, schemes, and dreams. He talked with his grandfather, Roby, for several minutes, and we ended the call as we always did … by saying, "I love you."

The next night, Roby's TV was on in the living room, and we were having a delightful visit when my cell phone rang. I stepped into the other room to answer it.

"Hello," I said, "this is Sherry."

"Hello," the female voice said on the other end of the phone. "This is the Orange County Sheriff's Department. Do you have a son named Brett Hobbs?"

The world seemed to stop. My heart felt as though it, too, had just stopped beating. I sat down and breathed deeply. "YYYeees," I said slowly. "Why, what's the matter?" I braced myself. An accident? A fight? A re-arrest? A slew of possibilities filtered through my head, except for the one thing she said next.

"I regret to inform you that your son has taken his own life. I'm afraid that he shot himself in the head while lying in his bed. I'm so sorry to have to tell you, Mrs. Hobbs."

Scene 11
Trying to Breathe

Mike and I flew home the following day in a daze, sobbing and holding each other as we wandered through the terminal, lost in our own thoughts. I called my sister from the airport, and we cried together, still not believing that it had really happened.

When we entered the house, it felt as though we were walking into a nightmare. Nothing felt real. We spoke with his friend Todd, who'd been there that night, and Kristy, who had rushed to the house the next day when Todd called her. He was distraught and sat holding his head in his hands. He told us that nothing seemed out of the ordinary the night before. Brett had ordered pizza, they drank a few beers, and they played a couple games of pool. After a while, Brett said he was going upstairs to bed.

Todd informed us that he soon fell asleep on the couch and didn't hear anything until the house cleaners woke him the following morning after they'd gone into Brett's room to clean. They found him lying face up on his bed, the gun on the floor below his outstretched right hand, blood splattered on the mirrored closet door. Todd called the police, and the room was roped off with crime scene tape.

The following is an email Mike wrote to friends and relatives two days after Brett's suicide:

Sunday, June 8, 2008

It goes without saying that this is the most difficult letter I have ever had to write. My preference, in fact, is to speak directly to each of you, but forgive me because I cannot get the words out at this time.

I am writing to you all to report what is an unbelievable tragedy for Sherry, me, and all who knew and loved our son. Our only child, Brett Michael Hobbs, died Friday, June 6, 2008. Brett took his own life while Sherry and I were in Indiana, attending to my father's health issues.

Brett was a gifted communicator, intelligent, outgoing, friendly, and very funny, especially when feeling well. He was also very knowledgeable in a wide variety of areas—an absolute information junkie—CNN, History Channel, politics, and anything that had to do with our planet and the creatures that live on it. If he heard it, he would never forget it. He had an IQ of 135.

That said, life was difficult for him. Early on, we learned that he had dyslexia and had attention deficit issues. Getting extra help and tutoring while in grade school made a difference. However, as he entered high school and had to attend special classes, he started feeling inferior and withdrew from formal education—ultimately getting a GED. From this point on, other psychological issues began emerging, the worst, of course, being depression.

Since his early twenties, he had been in hand-to-hand combat with depression. Brett was manic-depressive. He hated taking the medications—how they made him feel and, at times, look—but he took them. He needed the meds to exist for the last several years. Still, his mood swings were constant and worrisome for all. As he said, he just wanted to "be normal." And not to have the "weird feelings and thoughts." Knowing how much he loved his boys and his family, we did not—and could not—have envisioned his final alternative. May he truly rest in peace.

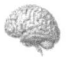

Going about our lives after that was like trying to walk in molasses. I felt as if I were in a trance. We just went through the motions, putting one foot in front of the other and pushing forward. The whirling thoughts in our brains consumed us separately. We had never discussed our feelings or shared the self-doubts we felt with each other. It was something that we needed to process individually.

I remembered Brett had recently told me, when talking about his impending prison sentence, *"You know, Mom, I've thought of suicide."*

He had said that before, and I'd always said, "But you'd never do that, right?"

And he had always agreed. *"I could never do that to my family."*

But this time, I didn't say the words, "But you'd never do that, right?" because the answer seemed so obvious, and I didn't need confirmation one more time. Did he take my silence for agreement? *Could I have prevented this horrible choice if I had only reminded him of his promise?* Over and over, that thought penetrated my brain, keeping me from sleep.

Thoughts and feelings swirled through my brain like air in a wind tunnel, consuming me with guilt, regret, and self-recrimination. The "what ifs" played in my head like a recording loop. *What if Brett had had a sibling? What if we had stayed in San Diego? What if we had insisted that he continue to attend regular high school?* These thoughts sang out endlessly in my head for weeks, months, and forever.

I tried to remind myself that we made the best decisions we could with the information we had at the time, but that never stopped the parade of questions and alternative scenarios that I'd created in my head. Was Mike plagued with the same kind of thoughts? We had never discussed those things because there were no answers, only mind-numbing questions that flitted unfettered forever through our brains.

Mike did tell me that he had found a gun in his safe in the office a week before we left for Indiana. It was *the* gun, as it turned out. He was shocked and confronted Brett about it at the time. Brett told him he was holding it for a friend who was selling it, and he promised his dad that it would be gone the next day. I'm sure Mike must have thought, *Could I have prevented Brett from killing himself if I had taken the gun away?*

The week after we had returned from Indiana, there was a flurry of activity—so many decisions and arrangements needed to be made. My family flew in from around the country to support and hold us up. Friends came from far and near, many staying all day, bringing everything from soup to quiet strength. There were over two hundred people at Brett's memorial service and celebration of life.

Then suddenly, it was over, and everyone went home. We had only his ashes and memories to hold on to. There was nothing more to do to keep us busy. We had to somehow pick up and continue our lives.

Mike went right back to work, and I followed a short time later. Both of us needed the distraction of plunging back into the minutia of our jobs. We needed to think about something other than our son, his decision to end his life, the heartbreaking fact that we would never see him again, and that his sons now eleven, ten, and nine, would grow up without him.

Barely two months later, fellow employees at Novellus had rushed Mike to the ER on two separate occasions, suspecting a heart attack, but doctors diagnosed him with panic–anxiety attacks. When he returned to work, Mike was tentative and lacked the confidence he had always had in abundance.

Steve told me years later that he kept telling the investors who were pressuring him to get the company up and running that Mike was still reeling from the death of his son. "This is an extremely talented man ... an incredible strategic thinker," he'd told them, trying to give Mike time to recover, process his grief, and snap back into the person he knew.

But investors are not patient people. And, as it turned out, more time would not have helped Mike anyway. Something in Mike's brain had died along with Brett. Mike discovered that while he read and studied the new information about pharmaceuticals and the trials needed to get them to market, he couldn't retain it. He couldn't learn it. He couldn't remember it. It wouldn't stick in his brain. Or, if it did, he couldn't access it.

Shortly before Christmas, Steve fired him ... just nine months after he'd offered him the position and six months after Brett's death. Little did we know then, but our lives were on the verge of a permanent major transformation. We were unwittingly on our way to a new chapter in our lives in a new place called Dementialand. We were sixty-one years old.

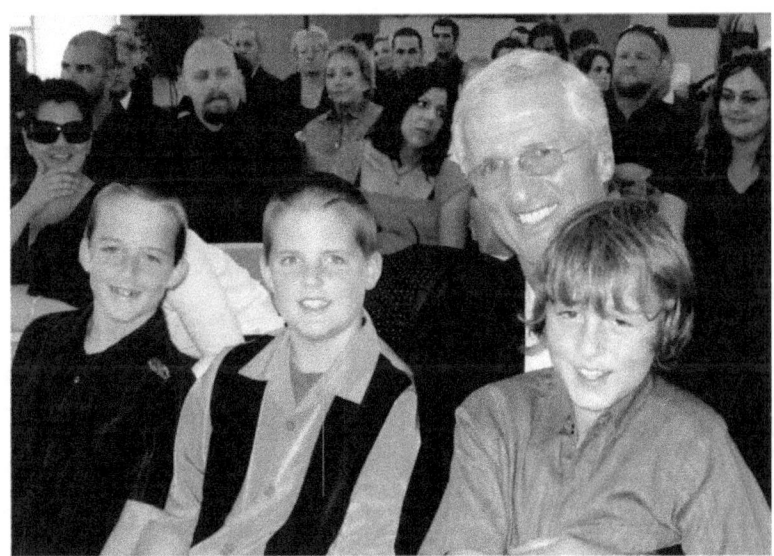

*Grandad trying to keep the boys upbeat and distracted at
their dad's memorial*

Scene 12

2008–2016: Strolling Down Main Street to FrontierWorld

When you wander down Main Street and first enter FrontierWorld, the atmosphere is cloudy and nothing is visible yet. You don't even realize you are in Dementialand, let alone FrontierWorld. That is because FrontierWorld can only be seen in retrospect once you enter the gates of AdventureWorld. Then, like Dorothy entering OZ, you see it in Technicolor if you look over your shoulder. We had entered FrontierWorld. We just didn't know it yet.

I am sure Steve agonized over letting Mike go. He was a close friend. Steve knew that Mike had suffered a devastating, crippling loss—his only child. But as president of the company, Steve was responsible to investors for building a successful business. When he had hired Mike as the chief operating officer, he entrusted him with establishing the process for conducting clinical trials, but Mike was unable to move forward. He was uncharacteristically stuck.

Steve had no doubt that the Mike he knew was up to the job. He believed in Mike and his abilities when he'd offered him the position. But Mike was not the man he once was, and no one knew why. I'm sure it became quickly apparent to everyone at Novellus that Mike was struggling to develop a protocol and act as a confident leader. He couldn't perform the job he was hired to do.

As Mike and I drifted into 2009, unsure of the trajectory of our lives, I threw myself into work and executed my stepfather's estate—he died in 2007—and my mother's. Mother had passed away in November, five months after Brett died. At eighty-two, the cause of her death was congestive heart failure, but it was complicated by the dementia she'd had for at least the last five years and probably much longer. She had spent her final year living with Cathe and Tom, enjoying a peaceful and happy existence.

On weekends, I busied myself with selling their home in Falls Church and distributing their property between her four children, according to their wills.

Out of work, Mike took his social security early at sixty-two and began working part-time with my brother, Derreck, managing some weight loss products that required minimal effort or new education but added a bit of income.

We had put the house up for sale, but after the 2008 global financial crisis, we watched our home's price drop precipitously from its highest valuation just the year before to rock bottom. To finance our son's short-lived carpet cleaning business, we had borrowed all the equity in the home, and eventually, the price of the house fell below the mortgaged amount. The bank agreed to a short sale, accepting less than what was owed. Mike's credit card debts and the loss of his income forced him to file for bankruptcy. We hired a clever attorney who was able to separate me financially from his bankruptcy, but our life felt like a beach house toppled by a tsunami wave train.

The next couple of years were a whirlwind of frantic activity and a blur like a video stuck on fast forward. Mike was unemployed for the first time in our lives, and our income suddenly dropped by two-thirds.

Fortunately, my mother had left me a small inheritance we could use as a down payment for a new home. However, the next house would need to be much smaller and require us to leave high-cost Southern California, where we had lived for the past thirty years. This meant not only moving away from longtime friends but also our three grandsons, with whom we were very close. This was extremely difficult for me, as my emotional ties to them and Southern California were strong. This was home.

Eventually, I yielded to Mike's practicality and slowly released the heartstrings that tied me to the state. He convinced me that the circumstances we'd found ourselves in left us with no other choice. At age sixty-three, we needed to rebuild our lives elsewhere. I let my company know that I would be relocating, and they agreed I could work from home, wherever home ended up being.

As I think back, Mike must have realized after taking the new job and studying the needed information that he was having trouble learning what had once come so easily. He must have been worried for some time, and I imagine Steve must have discussed it with him before he let him go.

However, Mike mentioned no concerns to me about his difficulty learning or the possibility of losing his job until dinner that fateful night, the week before it happened. And I never thought about the dinner confession Mike had made to me about having trouble learning or equating that inability with memory loss until years later. Looking back, with the benefit of hindsight, that was the first time there was any issue with Mike's memory, although I think that the actual onset of dementia was months earlier—the day we had learned that Brett was dead.

If Mike was worried about memory loss, he never allowed himself a minute to mourn the job itself. It was done, and he would pick up and move ahead as he always had when encountering setbacks. He never missed a beat after losing his job, most of our livelihood, and our home. We'd start over somewhere else ... somewhere warm, somewhere west, and somewhere less expensive to live. He was, as usual, positive and upbeat. And I, as usual, was with him.

After mulling over several relocation options, we'd decided to move to Henderson, Nevada, where houses were less expensive and my sister Cathe and her husband, Tom, lived. Plus, it was only a four-to-five-hour drive from Southern California or an hour's flight. I told myself we wouldn't be that far from the grandsons, who were now preteens and had friends and weekend activities to keep them busy. I rationalized that they didn't have to be with their grandparents every weekend, even if their grandmother needed to be with them.

While I continued to work, Mike busied himself finding homes for us to look at and mortgage companies that would take a chance on us. We drove back and forth to Henderson frequently and finally settled on a small, three-bedroom, one-story home with a pool on the same short cul-de-sac where Cathe and Tom lived. I reluctantly dragged myself, along with downsized possessions and furniture, the 269 miles to Henderson, Nevada. This was, by my count, the twenty-seventh time I had moved in my lifetime.

By the time Cathe and Tom's son, Devon, and his family moved in across the street from them a year later, our family had established quite the neighborhood compound. We owned one-fifth of the houses on the short street called Bearclaw Terrace. I mused that our family occupied one claw on that bear's paw, amusing only myself.

Mike became a regular at Home Depot, enjoying relative fame where, like *Cheers*, everyone knew his name. He loved decorating and picked out most of the outdoor lighting and home improvement items. He visited there daily, selecting the myriad things needed in a new home.

He supervised the renovation and updating of the kitchen and bathrooms. With the radically lower house payment and utilities, we were managing well on my salary and the smaller amount Mike brought in. He was his usual happy-go-lucky self. I didn't suspect then, for one minute, that there was anything wrong with his brain. But of course, Ratt had, in fact, burrowed in and was slowly destroying neurons—the nerve cells that send and receive signals from the brain.

Our first year in Henderson, 2010, was a particularly glorious and triumphant year for Mike in that the Butler Bulldogs, our college team on which he had played as a freshman and sophomore, had earned a spot in the NCAA basketball tournament. The team was exceptional, and we watched and rooted for them every game on television during March Madness, cheering them on to each subsequent victory, connecting, and sharing the excitement with college friends who were spread out around the country.

When the Bulldogs made it into the Sweet Sixteen bracket, this offered us a very welcome distraction. We went on the road each weekend and physically followed them to every game, culminating in the Final Four tournament in Indianapolis. We'd traveled to each new city as they competed, meeting up with old friends from Butler.

Spending so much time with Bob and Carol Moeller was particularly gratifying. Bob, Mike's best friend who had also played on the basketball team with him, had been fighting colon cancer for the last couple of years. They flew out to join us for every game, and we extended each weekend to vacation in the host city.

The tournament ended in Indianapolis in a heart-stopping, nail-biting, last-minute shot by Butler's Gordon Hayward that bounced off the rim, with Duke squeaking by the Butler Bulldogs 59–61. We watched that last game sitting courtside at Lucas Oil Stadium, six miles from Butler University where Mike and Bob had played basketball and we'd all met forty-three years before.

We missed and mourned our son, but we both seemed to be getting on with life. I thought about Brett daily whenever I saw a black, Ford pickup truck, someone on a Suzuki motorcycle, or a heavily tattooed, young man, and I assumed Mike did as well. Brett came to me frequently in dreams and still does. Mike and I didn't talk much about him when we were together, but we often watched the many videos I had created from years of photos, particularly the one we showed at Brett's Celebration of Life. It was bittersweet.

We also felt and saw Brett in each of our three grandsons, whom I initially felt wrenched away from. But instead of weekend visits, the boys became frequent fliers on Southwest Airlines and visited us three times a year—a week in the summers, during the Christmas holidays, and during spring breaks.

Mike and I joined "Fill-a-Seat," which, for a nominal annual fee, gave members access to free tickets to many Las Vegas shows that hadn't sold out, and we took full advantage. Most shows were second tier but not second-rate. All were entertaining. When the boys visited, we took them to see magicians and family-friendly comedians, which they loved. Las Vegas had much to explore and offered lots of things to do beyond the famed gambling casinos.

We discovered that Las Vegas had a small but vibrant theater community, so we immediately sought it out and bought season tickets to two of them, continuing our Sunday matinee habit. We had always loved indie movies and foreign films, so we regularly drove the half hour north to Summerlin to attend the only theater that showed them. The Las Vegas cultural scene was in its infancy but growing steadily. Symphony Park was named in downtown Las Vegas in 2008, and in 2012, the Smith Center for Performing Arts opened its world-class doors.

During these first few years in Henderson, we had frequently traveled to Indiana to visit Mike's dad, Roby, who was now happily ensconced in the assisted living facility. We would fly into Indianapolis, stay with the Moellers for the weekend, and then drive to Centerville to visit Roby before returning home.

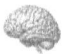

My position with Ameritas required me to travel a couple of weeks out of the month, and I loved that part of the job. Of course, I always loved to travel, and meeting the people I'd worked with in person was a bonus. It was also "me time" for a couple of evenings, usually every other week. After a day of visiting customers, I would look forward to dinner at the hotel, a glass or two of wine, and then crawl into bed with a good book. Many longtime customers became friends, and I enjoyed spending an occasional evening at dinner with them.

Each time I flew out, Mike dropped me off at the airport and picked me up after the return flight. I loved my job, and Mike was his usual upbeat, gregarious self, perfectly content with working part-time, playing golf on the weekends, and chauffeuring me to the airport. He also worked out by shooting baskets in pickup games at the community center for the first few years until an old shoulder injury permanently sidelined him.

When I was not traveling, Mike and I enjoyed Henderson's new, slower-paced environment, quickly resuming our California lifestyle of golf on weekends on the many courses that the Las Vegas area boasted. Henderson offered the bonus of having a proliferation of public courses that were well maintained and with substantially lower green fees than California links. We played frequently with Cathe and Tom, went out to dinner regularly, and skied when it was in season, traveling to one of the many ski resorts in Utah or back to Mammoth Mountain in California. Life was good, and we were still having fun, even in the sweltering Nevada sun.

If his dementia began in 2008, then during these first few years in Henderson, Mike and I were in FrontierWorld, the first park in Dementialand. FrontierWorld encompasses the first three stages on the GDS. A kind of pre-early dementia.

These were enjoyable and mostly unremarkable years because we were unaware of where we were. We thought we were still in Normaland, as the slide is such a slow and gradual drop that it's almost impossible to know that you had arrived in FrontierWorld until you land in AdventureWorld and look back up to where you were.

I have since learned that those first three stages of dementia are so mild, they are virtually unrecognizable at the time. With a couple of lost words here and there, people assume it's stress, normal aging, or a "senior moment." As people age, everyone forgets where they put their keys from time to time or the name of someone they'd just met. And moments are, by definition, fleeting and easy to forget and dismiss. Aren't they? They are normal—unless they are not—and you later find yourself in Adventureland.

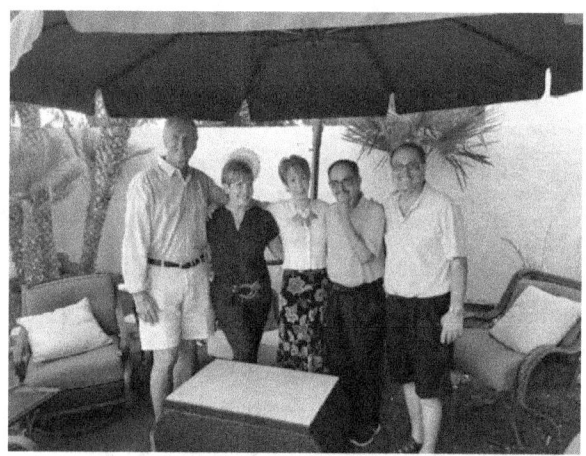

*Mike, Cathe, me, John (Tom's brother), and Tom.
Dinner at Cathe and Tom's house.*

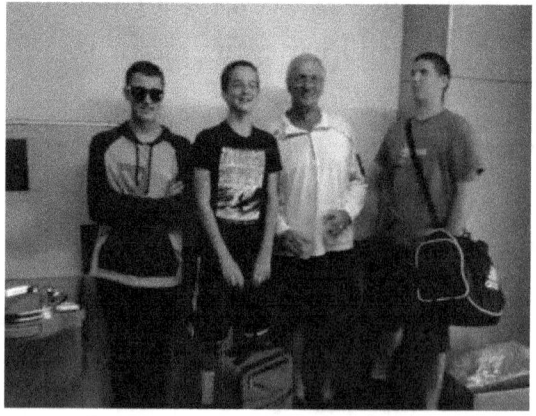

The jet setters visit us in Henderson

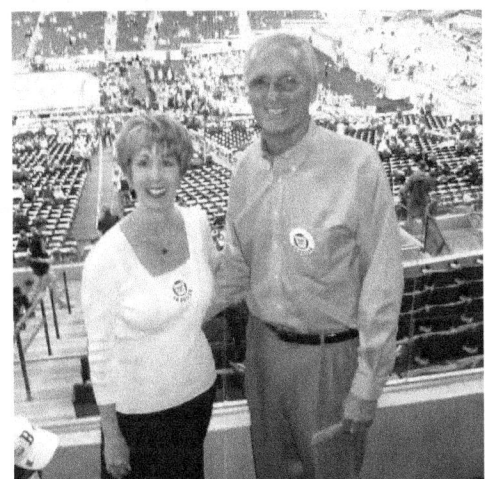

*At Lucas Oil Stadium to see the final NCAA game
Butler v Duke*

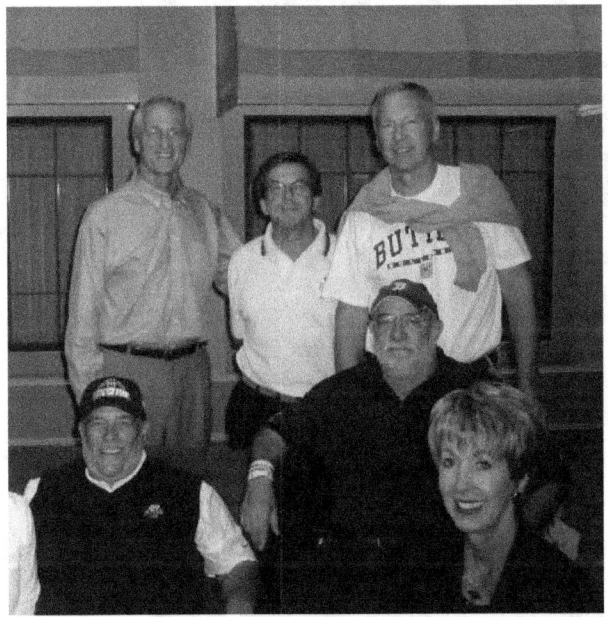

With fellow Butler friends

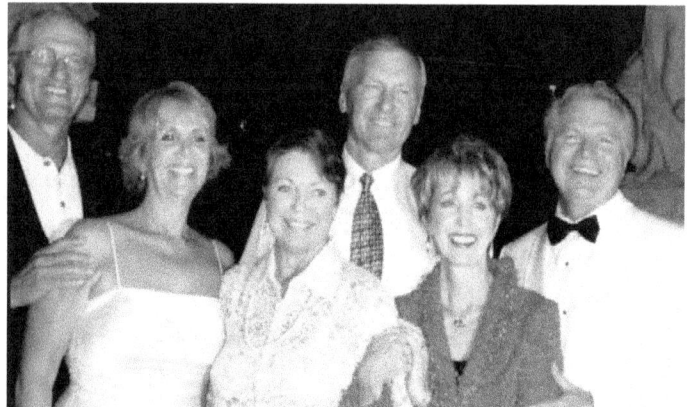

Celebrating a milestone with our longtime Butler friends

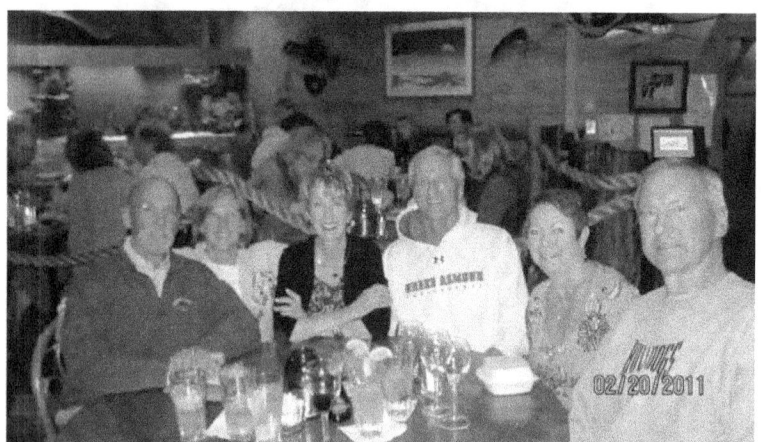

Pre-final NCAA game. 2010 Butler v Duke

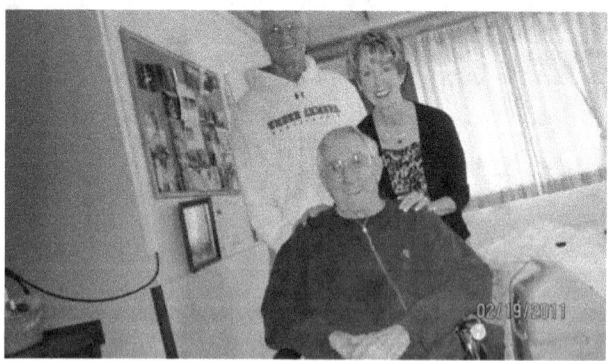

Visiting with Roby in his new digs

Scene 13

And Bijou Makes Three ... in FrontierWorld

In the fall of 2011, Mike and I were preparing to fly to Maui, Hawaii, for a week of golf and culinary indulgences. The day before our flight, I stopped to get a manicure. On my way home, I passed a sign in a Puppyland store that boasted PUPPY SALE in big, red letters. Mike and I had talked about adding another dog to our family and decided against it. Or he had.

Our last beloved canine, a Bichon Frisé named Mr. Blue, passed away from kidney failure shortly before we'd left Southern California. We told ourselves this was not the time to bring a new puppy into the home. We traveled frequently, and dogs were family members requiring much time and attention. So we were definitely not going to get one anytime soon. Plus, we were headed to Maui for a week of golf. This was just not the right time. I thought, *Well, it certainly can't hurt to look.*

I parked the car and entered the store, glancing briefly at the signs on the cages. A clerk approached. "Would you like to see one of the puppies?" she asked.

"No thanks. My husband is allergic to dander, and we have to have a non-shedding dog. I was looking for a Bichon Frisé, but I see you don't have any." I turned to walk out.

"True, but we have a Zuchon. That's half Shih Tzu and half Bichon, and they are also hypoallergenic. Step into this booth, and I'll show her to you." *Well,* I thought again, *it can't hurt to look,* and I sat on the bench in the small enclosure.

Then she brought in the cutest puppy I had ever seen. She was white with black ears and forehead, a black splotch on her back, a white-and-black tail, and a black rear end that looked like she was wearing a pair of black, lace panties. The back of her tail that curled up and pointed at her backside was black, matching the panties, and the front side of the tail was white, matching her back.

As the sales clerk put her down on my lap, the little dog stood on her tiny legs and furiously licked my face as if to say, *pick me, pick me!* "I have to talk to my husband," I told the woman. "I'll be back."

Mike and I were running errands that afternoon, and I asked him to go into the shopping center under some pretense. "Just park the car. I want to show you something," I said.

He glanced toward the store as he exited the car, spotting the ominous sign PUPPY SALE. "No way!" he asserted.

"Just come in a minute," I pleaded, pulling him by the hand. "I just want to show you something." He sighed. I signaled the clerk, and we both entered the small booth. As she walked in, latching the door behind her, she handed the puppy to Mike, and immediately, the sly dog began licking his face. He turned his head and glared at me.

"She's quite the little saleswoman," he said snidely. And that was it. After calling my sister to ensure they would foster her for a week, we left, loaded with containers, food, toys, and a little puppy I dubbed Bijou, French for jewel. I also refer to her as The Love Dog (TLD) for her propensity to kiss everyone, and she is.

Six months later, while I was walking in the park behind our house with Bijou leading the way, a sudden, horrific thunderstorm appeared out of nowhere, creating a pounding rainstorm complete with lightning and thunder. *From what horrible monster was this unholy noise emanating,* Bijou must have thought, and she slipped out of her harness and raced through the pounding rain toward home and safety. I ran after her but could not keep up with the terrified, little animal.

It was almost impossible to see anything through the blinding torrents of water. When I arrived home, she was nowhere around. I got in the car and slowly drove through the neighborhood, calling her name. Eventually, we discovered her under the bed in Cathe's home, which is closer to the park than ours, and of course, it was her early foster home. She had apparently run through their open garage door and raced up the stairs to hide under their bed, sheltering from the angry storm monster. Of course, she later developed PTSD and has been terrified of all loud noises ever since. She cowered behind the toilet bowl, draping herself around the porcelain base like a mink stole whenever she smelled rain in the air.

Bijou is a delightfully entertaining dog. She has the same tendency to run laps around the dining room table as our two Bichon Frisés had. Some call it the Zoomies; we call it the Puppy 500. But Bijou adds a twist. She runs a few laps in one direction, grabs a squeaky toy, tosses it into the air, and reverses her course. She does this for about five minutes, then stops, smiles like a Cheshire cat, and waits for her just compensation like any virtuoso performer. In her case, it is a chicken-wrapped rawhide stick, which she gnaws clean in about thirty seconds and then spits out the stick, quite proud of herself.

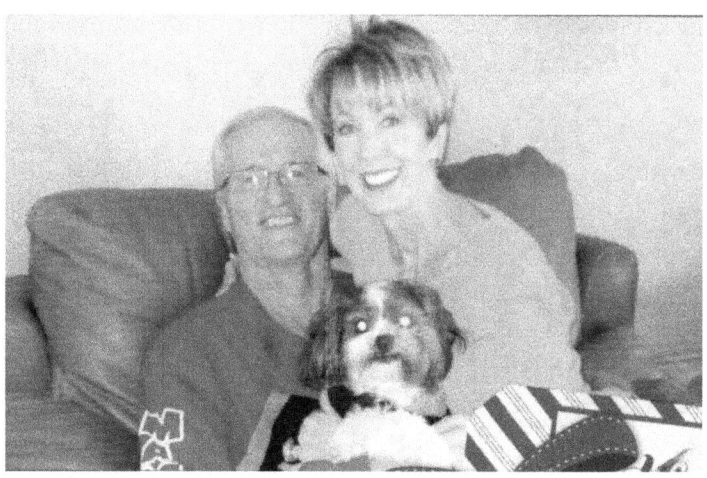

Our nuclear family in Henderson

Scene 14

The Rickety Bridge from FrontierWorld to AdventureWorld

Stage 3 - Global Deterioration Scale (GDS) / Reisberg Scale			
Diagnosis	Stage	Signs and Symptoms	Expected Duration of Stage
Pre-dementia	Stage 3: Mild Cognitive Decline	– Increased forgetfulness – Slight difficulty concentrating – Decreased work performance – Gets lost more frequently – Difficulty finding right words – Loved ones begin to notice	The average duration of this stage is between 2 years and 7 years.

Stage 3 Table: Applicable to Scenes 14 through 17

Time seemed to fly by. We had lived in Henderson for two years. We were happy, enjoying life with thrice-yearly visits from our grandsons and frequent trips back to California. We vacationed in Hawaii and skied in Utah and Mammoth. Everything seemed normal. Mike now occasionally used the wrong word or forgot something he ordinarily would not have. Just senior moments, I thought.

Mike's dad passed away in September 2012, and we flew back to Indiana for a week to take care of the funeral arrangements. We stayed in Indianapolis with Carol Moeller. Bob was now in a nursing home with end-stage colon cancer, and we'd spent what would be his last week of life visiting with him. He passed away shortly after we left. Mike typed a beautiful eulogy for the funeral, recalling his best friend and fraternity brother and the many good times the four of us had shared since college. As Mike's eulogy was read, smiles and laughs punctuated the air and softened the tears shed. Mike's detailed remembrances and well-written tribute gave no hint of any brain impairment.

In the spring of 2013, it had been a little over five years since Mike lost his job and three years since we had relocated to Nevada. On a beautiful spring day in Henderson, we made a tee time to play golf with my sister and Tom, as we frequently had. Mike drove the three of us in his truck and dropped us off, along with our golf bags, at the bag drop as he usually did, and the three of us went inside to pay for the round in the pro shop. Normally, Mike would then park the truck and join the group inside. He joined us inside but apparently had forgotten to park the truck.

When we returned to the pro shop after four and a half hours of golf, it shocked us to learn that he'd left the truck on and running for the entire time out front under the portico. While Cathe and Tom teased him good-naturedly and tried to laugh it off, I quietly fought back tears. This was big. And this was not the first time he had forgotten something he ordinarily would have easily remembered. I was now frightened about what the future held for him—for us—as this wasn't just a momentary memory lapse, and it was becoming a pattern.

In 2014, our lives remained busy and largely unchanged. Mike continued to have memory issues or lost words from time to time, but mostly, everything still seemed normal. We drove to California one weekend to visit grandsons and good friends, and surprisingly, Mike had difficulty finding his way around and locating houses we'd lived in and restaurants we had frequented for thirty years.

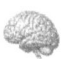

When our brother-in-law, Tom, retired from teaching, he and Mike joined two senior bowling leagues—one on Monday mornings and one on Wednesday afternoons. John, Tom's brother, and Joanne, a friend, rounded out their team. Mike still loved to golf but complained that the shoulder injury caused him problems swinging a golf club. He had quit shooting baskets, and golf became less frequent. Bowling was now his favorite pastime, and he competed ferociously. He had a solid 160 average.

Our grandsons continued to visit three times a year, and we always ensured they were well entertained. Besides gambling and shows, the Las Vegas area offered a surprising number of other activities, including a small, local ski resort about forty-five minutes north of the city. With only a couple of ski lifts and a handful of runs, it was an excellent spot for the boys to learn. They took skiing lessons and were eager to go again. We told them we'd take them to Mammoth the following year for an authentic ski experience, and we did. They were hooked.

Dave Andrews, a friend from Butler who lives in Salt Lake City, owned a second home in Overton, Nevada, about forty-five minutes east of Henderson, where he and his wife kept a large stable of four-wheelers. Dave knew all of the trails and local lore. They had hosted us numerous times for a different kind of adventure, and we took the boys, who were thrilled with the desert experience. We would spend the day riding the four-wheelers, picnicking, and exploring the caves and petroglyphs in the Valley of Fire.

My brother, Derreck, who liked scuba diving, had joined TradeWinds, a timeshare-like cruise club for people who wanted to sail, scuba dive, snorkel, or just plain party like a rock star aboard a yacht. He invited Mike and me on a week's trip through the British Virgin Islands, and we were delighted to accept and accompany him.

We paid our "all-inclusive" charge, which covered all of the food and drinks for the week, and Mike and I immersed ourselves in the crystal-clear waters of the Caribbean Ocean. The myriad islets, cays, and rocks around the major islands are magical places to discover and explore. It was exhilarating when we were under sail, feeling the wind in our hair and watching the ocean waves undulate endlessly. I enjoyed lying on the deck under a canopy, slathered in sunscreen, reading books I had brought or found in the small cabin library. Once we anchored, I swam or snorkeled with Mike. It was a real vacation from reality.

On one seemingly magical day, dolphins playfully followed the boat. Then Captain Chris put down the anchor, and the highly intelligent mammals jumped and dove, enthralling us with a performance worthy of a Cirque du Soleil spectacular. As we drifted or sailed along, Mike, in his element, sat in a sportsman's chair at the yacht's bow, soaking up the sun and watching the ocean and playful animals. Life was good, and Mike's marriage vow to entertain me was upheld once again.

Mammoth had received a big dump of snow that winter, so we drove to the Sierra Nevada mountain range for a three-day ski trip. Except for Europe, where I was more comfortable, Mike was always in charge of planning, and this trip was no exception. He packed our ski gear, arranged for the condo, and drove us the 323 miles to Mammoth Lakes.

The day I knew that leaving the packing to Mike was no longer possible was after we had arrived at the condo. As we geared up to ski the following morning, we discovered he had brought our bowling balls instead of our ski helmets. We had a good laugh, with mine a little less mirthful than his. Okay, the carry bags looked very similar, but this was not something he would typically mix up. *How did he not notice the weight difference when he loaded thirty pounds of bowling balls into the car?*

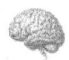

Because we wanted to keep sharing adventures with our grandsons and exposing them to travel, Mike and I had promised each of them several years earlier that we would take them on a trip to Europe after graduating from high school. Davin, the oldest, was first. He had planned to enlist in the army and serve two years before attending college.

We drove to Southern California in June for Davin's high school graduation, and in the fall, we took him on a European adventure. Since France is my favorite foreign country, and I knew Paris so well, having lived there, it was an easy choice. Besides, Mike was now a certified Francophile. We couldn't wait to show Davin Gay Paree, Versailles, and Normandy.

In September 2015, before Davin left for basic training, we flew to Paris on an extraordinary excursion. Can you imagine my delight in showing my oldest grandson around France's glamorous and historic places? Mike had a great time as well. He was also delighted to share the experience with his grandson and me. We biked around the City of Lights, spent a day at the Louvre, hiked up to Sacré-Coeur, and had dinner in Montmartre. We strolled around the square, watching artists paint and draw as tourists and locals milled about—a chromesthesia of sound, color, and movement like the swirling skirts of Mexican folk dancers.

We took a train to Versailles the following day and biked around the city. Stocking up on baguettes, cheese, meat, fruit, and wine at an outdoor market, we picnicked on the banks of the lake facing the palace, toured the magnificent interior, and visited Marie Antoinette's peasant village. During the many times I had visited Versailles, I'd never seen the faux city the young queen had built so she could play house with her courtiers and imagine how the peasants lived. *No wonder the French Revolution occurred,* I thought.

Toward the end of the week, we took the high-speed train north to Normandy, and Davin marveled at the American Cemetery, exquisite memorial gardens, and D-Day beaches. It was a beautiful, warm day with a gentle breeze as we stood on the expansive beach.

Our French tour guide, Alain, was passionate and visibly emotional about what had happened there in June 1944, almost exactly seventy-one years before, and described in detail how the brave Americans liberated

France. He especially wanted Davin, a young man who was going into the army, to appreciate the sacrifices the Americans had made and the heartfelt gratitude that he and other French people felt for their extraordinary efforts.

He took him aside, and they stood on the sand. I watched Alain tilt his head, look deep into Davin's eyes, and pound his fist against his palm. He drew in the sand with a stick, pointing at the ocean where thousands of young soldiers—most of them Davin's age—waded to shore under heavy machine gunfire. Then he turned and pointed at the cement bunkers from where the Germans sprayed them relentlessly with bullets. Twenty-nine thousand men had lost their lives, and 137,000 suffered injuries in the twenty-seven days of the Normandy Invasion, a staggering statistic.

After touring the bunkers and stepping into the immense craters left by bombs, Davin sat inside the beautiful chapel alone to reflect on the events and sacrifices of the thousands of men who'd died there during WWII. I'm sure it held special significance to him as he was days away from being inducted into the army.

I can only remember one incident on this trip that concerned me about Mike's declining memory. Back in Paris one evening, Mike was sick with a cold and begged off dinner because he wasn't feeling well and wanted to sleep. Since the Eiffel Tower was only a few blocks from our hotel, I told Mike we'd planned to stop on our way back since Davin wanted to see it at night.

Leaving Mike to rest in the hotel room, Davin and I ventured out for dinner with my French friend, Odile. We took the Metro to the stop where she had suggested we meet her, ate dinner at a charming local bistro, and then headed to the Eiffel Tower. We rode the elevator to the top and stared at the glorious City of Lights. The view, of course, was spectacular ... something to cross off his bucket list.

I was so caught up in the extraordinary moment with my grandson that I didn't realize how late it was. It was nearly midnight when we'd returned to the hotel, and Mike was frantic and panicky. He didn't remember what I had told him we were doing. He didn't know where we were or how to contact us. I apologized profusely and told myself this was a perfectly normal reaction. He was sick, he didn't speak French, and he had no phone with which to call me. *Of course, he would be distraught if we disappeared and he couldn't reach us,* I thought. But it was unlike him to be panicky.

When we had returned home to Henderson, more red flags from Dementialand started popping up, waving in the breeze, trying to get my attention. Mike's conversational skills were deteriorating, and he couldn't remember many things from the past. Occasionally, he even had trouble remembering some recent events and would ask me the same question several times.

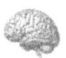

Bob and Pandy Roberts, close friends from our Butler days, lived near us in San Juan Capistrano when we lived in Laguna Hills. We watched each other's children grow up. They visited us several times over the five years since we had moved to Henderson, and Pandy suffered from early dementia. She was subsequently diagnosed with Alzheimer's and sadly passed away on November 21, 2015. It was jarring. Her decline and eventual death were rapid and precipitous. She was only sixty-eight years old.

Long planned, Mike and I headed to the British Virgin Islands for another yacht trip during Thanksgiving week. Our friends and neighbors, Mike and Brenda, joined us. Derreck and Suzanne had intended to come, but at the last minute, they had an emergency with their business and could not travel.

Mike was now more subdued around people, and those who had not known him beforehand could not have guessed he was ever "Mr. Personality." By the same token, they hadn't known him long enough or well enough to suspect dementia. But I did. His communication skills had vastly slowed, and he was no longer confident engaging with people he did not know well.

However, the two Mikes sat in easy chairs on the boat's bow, drank rum cocktails, and somehow managed to swap stories, apparently having a great time. I'm sure that the rum helped, at least as far as neighbor Mike being able to understand everything Mike Hobbs talked about. Brenda and I snorkeled and explored the islands while the two pirates enjoyed ho-ho-hijinks and a bottle of rum.

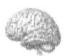

In May 2016, Mike, Sunneshine, and I flew to Missouri to see Davin graduate from basic training at Ft. Leonard Wood. It was a proud moment for all of us. We toured the fort and watched the graduates' parade, culminating in the evening graduation ceremony.

In July, we drove to Orange County to see our second grandson, Gavin, graduate from high school. We asked him if he wanted to go on his trip separately as Davin had, or if he would rather wait a year until Corben graduated when we could take both boys on their European adventure together. He wanted to go with Corben, and Corben also loved the idea. I set about planning another grand adventure with the grandsons for the following summer.

Since Davin had mustered out of the army and both he and Corben were going to start college in the fall, we decided to invite him as well. We also included their mom, Sunneshine, who had never been to Europe, and she was delighted to share the experience with her sons. Since Davin had already visited France, we wanted to take the group to Italy for this trip in June 2017 after Corben graduated. With just a week, I planned to show them Rome and Pompeii.

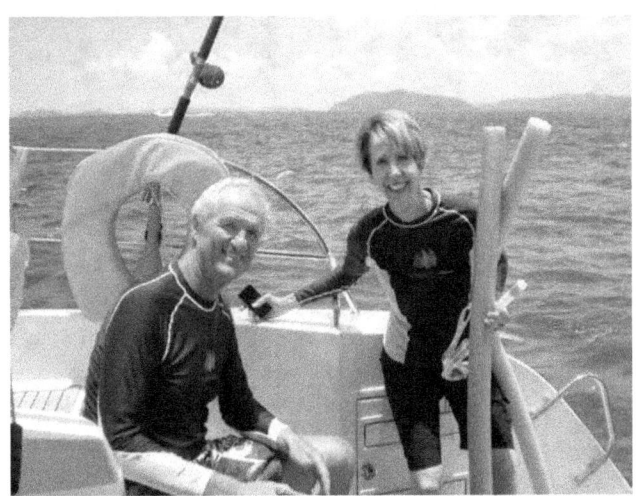

Snorkeling in the British Virgin Islands

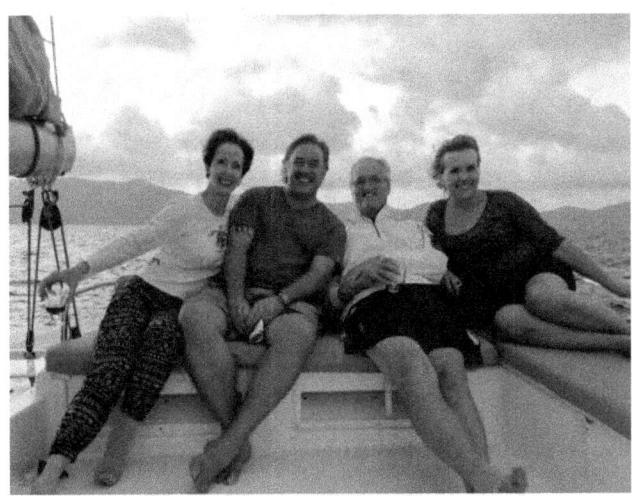

On the catamaran with brother Derreck

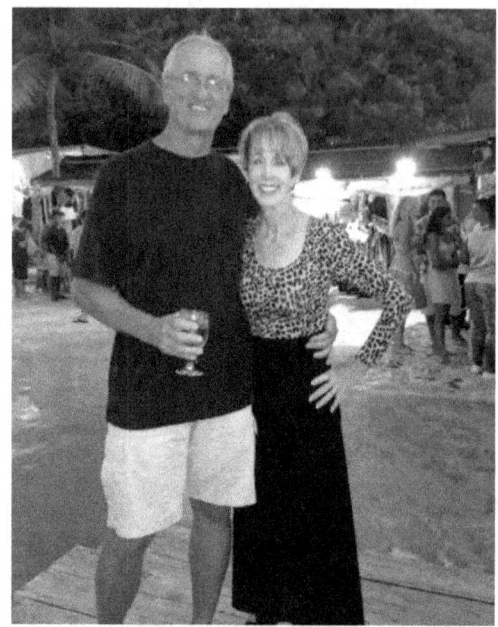

Dinner at the Soggy Dollar in Jost Van Dyke, BVI

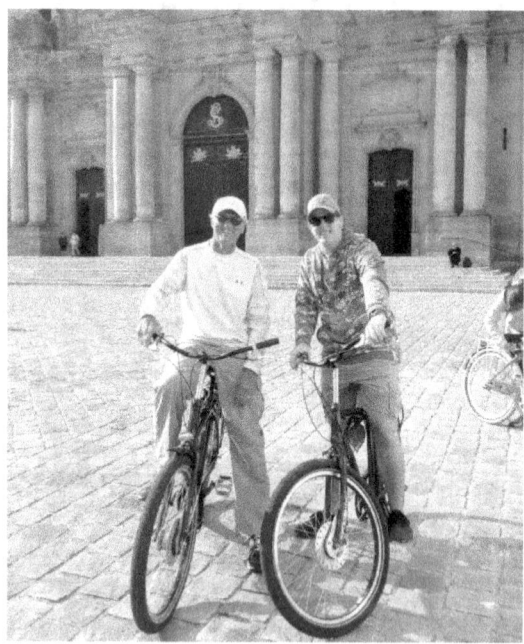

Touring Paris by bike with Davin

Scene 15

2017: Creating Episodic Memories

Mike began experiencing increasing memory loss and difficulty using certain words. He might say, "I put my glove on the wrong foot," or "I drove down the sled" instead of the street. Sometimes, he caught himself, and sometimes, he didn't. He was uncomfortable driving places he was unfamiliar with.

In March, I had a routine colonoscopy scheduled at an outpatient facility about a half hour from home. I set the GPS on my phone to guide us there. Mike drove us in his Ford Expedition and sat in the waiting room with me while I waited to be called. There was a McDonald's restaurant across the parking lot, and I suggested he walk over there during my procedure, get breakfast, then walk back and sit in the waiting room until they released me, no more than an hour and a half or so.

When I awoke in the recovery room, the nurses told me that they had paged Mike several times and that he didn't appear to be in the lobby. I called him on his cell phone and discovered, much to my surprise, that he had driven home. The McDonald's was closed for renovations, and he forgot that I was in surgery but somehow found his way back to the house. He had no idea where I was or how to return to the clinic. He had never learned to use GPS on his truck, and, of course, he only had a flip phone with no GPS on it, either—not that he could have used either one. I called Tom, who was walking off the golf course, and he came and retrieved me.

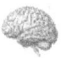

After Corben graduated in June, we set out on our grand and glorious Italian adventure. This trip included Rome and Pompeii, which had mesmerized me when I was just a year younger than Corben, and a brief but delightful stop in Sorento. Mike, a happy traveler, was, as always, content to let me take the lead in Europe. I booked the travel and tours and created the itinerary. I don't think anyone other than me detected anything seriously wrong with Granddad's communication ability. And maybe it was because we were all so busy seeing the sights.

On the last night in Rome, all three boys, who were now in their late teens and early twenties, got their first tattoo. They took the subway to a negozio di tatuaggi they had passed by one day, and the artist inscribed a plain, black tattoo—**VIVIMMVIII**—on the inside of their wrists. This was the date that their father had died, June 6, 2008, and they were in Rome on that anniversary, nine years later. So, of course, they thought it fitting to have the artist ink it in Roman numerals.

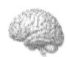

Mike and I turned seventy in August and September 2017 and had lived in Henderson for seven years. With each passing day, it became apparent that he was suffering from some kind of dementia. Besides forgetting how to get around in his truck, Mike was less confident about his abilities and needed help at home, forgetting where some things belonged and how to navigate life when he was by himself. He became nervous about staying alone overnight when I was out of town. His condition was such that my leaving on work trips became difficult for both of us. I knew that these incidents were not typical "senior moments." Whatever brain damage there was, it was slowly getting worse. I needed to pick a retirement date and let my company know soon.

One day, when I was busy working at home, Mike volunteered to drive my sister and Tom to the airport. It is about fifteen minutes from the house and a straight shot down one road that runs behind our house. He had made that trip hundreds of times, taking me to the airport and picking me up after my business trips. On this occasion, however, when he exited the airport, he made a wrong turn and got lost on the way home.

He pulled over and frantically called me. He was understandably panicky, as he had no idea where he was or how to find our house. I asked him to look for the street signs, pull into a nearby gas station or business, and tell me what the signs said. When I finally found him, he was very distraught and followed me home in his truck. I never had to have that talk about handing over the car keys. That ended his desire to drive anywhere alone.

He continued to drive his truck with me in the passenger seat for quick trips on familiar routes. Since most of our driving was within two miles of the house, I felt he was still up to the task. However, I noticed his reflexes were slowing, so I knew it was only a matter of time before I would need to take over the driving full time.

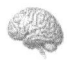

Many years before, Mike and I had purchased two timeshare weeks at The Palm Springs Tennis Club. Since moving to Henderson, we used them to meet the grandsons and Sunneshine for a week each November or December. It is only a forty-five-minute drive from their home, and we could celebrate an early Christmas with gift exchanges and a special dinner at the upscale, holiday-festive Spencer's Restaurant. It became a tradition.

This December, we invited good friends Richard and Susie Graham to join us for a few days before the boys arrived. Richard had been Mike's fraternity brother at Butler and my frequent bridge partner in the C-Club. We reconnected when we'd moved to California and bonded solidly after they lost one of their twin daughters to meningitis when she was a college student in San Diego. Susie had reluctantly retired in 2009 after thirty-eight years of teaching due to problems related to MS. She subsequently developed dementia but continued to play duplicate bridge until this year, when her longtime partner, whom she had tasked with delivering this message, kindly and lovingly advised that it was time for her to quit.

The four of us had a great time visiting and exploring the downtown Palm Springs area, but Susie insisted she wanted to ride bicycles, which the timeshare provided. Never particularly athletic, this didn't seem like a good idea to the rest of us. However, she persisted, and we all checked out bikes. Ten minutes and three falls later, we returned the bikes and played table shuffleboard in the game room. It was much safer. Shades of what was coming with Mike? I wondered.

Back at home, Mike and I enjoyed playing Scrabble in the afternoons. We had a large, wooden board with wood tiles that were easy to read and place. However, during games now, he sometimes lost focus and frequently asked about the spelling of common words. When he put down the tiles to form an intended word like LINE, he would mix up the order and place it as LNIE.

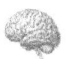

One of Mike's most endearing qualities is his tenaciousness about maintaining relationships no matter where we or our friends lived in the country. He called them frequently, checked in with them on Facebook, and planned trips to visit them or for us to take joint vacations together. He never let a friendship languish from neglect if he could help it.

Over the next few months, I found Mike had gradually lost the ability to look at his favorite sports websites or monitor the Facebook page he'd always enjoyed using to keep in touch with friends. The computer confounded him now, although he never mentioned it. He still carried an old-fashioned flip phone, which he only used to call me when needed.

Soon, I started paying some of the bills online while he continued to pay the ones that came by mail with a check. He had always managed the finances but began having increased difficulty paying the bills. He was not yet ready for me to do a complete takeover, but I closely monitored him, looking over his shoulder and standing in the shadows to ensure the bills got paid.

Next, I hired a financial planner who, like a Japanese, pearl-diving Ama, took a deep dive into our finances and upcoming retirement income, which included my 401(k) and pension with Ameritas, plus social security.

"You have enough," she said when she broke the surface for air, "to retire reasonably comfortably."

I felt better, but it was still terrifying to me. It felt like stepping off a cliff blindfolded and falling headfirst into a lake. Could I just give up my good income and job I loved? I had been with Ameritas for twenty years. Even at seventy, I wasn't ready to retire. However, Mike needed me. Once again, life's events gave me little choice. I gave the company six months' notice and told Ameritas I would retire on May 1st of the following year.

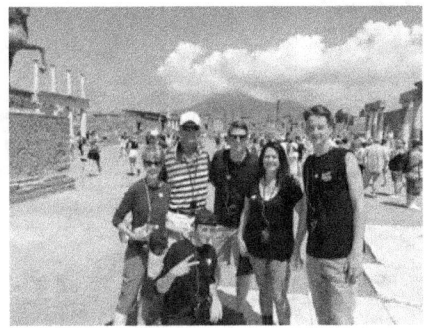

Pompeii with Mt. Vesuvius in background

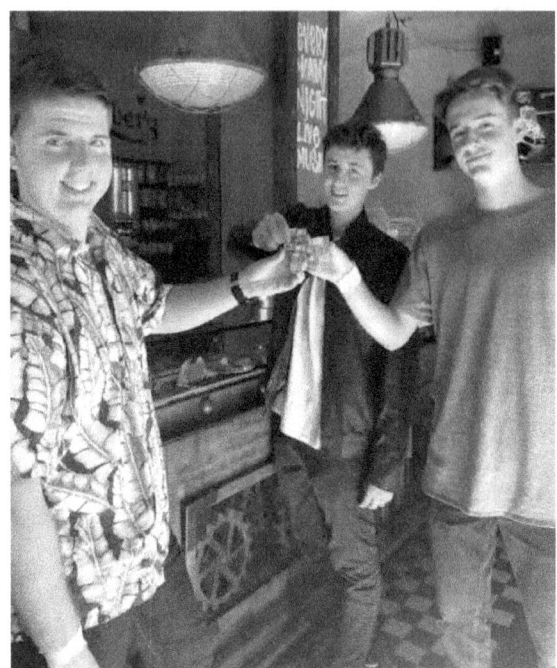

A toast to their dad

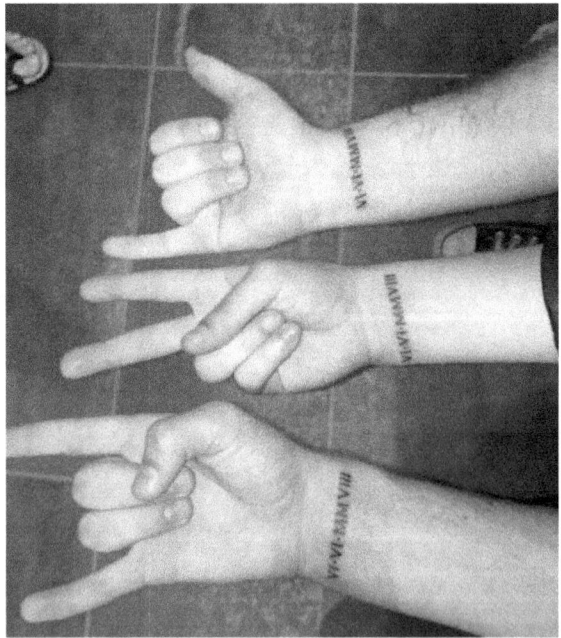

VIVIMMVIII. The anniversary of Brett's death in Rome

Scene 16

2018: The Diagnosis and the Gateway to Adventureland

Stage 4 - Global Deterioration Scale (GDS) / Reisberg Scale			
Diagnosis	Stage	Signs and Symptoms	Expected Duration of Stage
Early-stage	Stage 4: Moderate Cognitive Decline	– Difficulty concentrating – Forgets recent events – Cannot manage finances – Cannot travel alone to new places – Difficulty completing tasks – In denial about symptoms – Socialization problems: Withdraws from friends or family – Physician can detect cognitive problems	The average duration of this stage is 2 years.

Stage 4 Table: Applicable to Scenes 16 through 22

Mike and I both knew that we needed to get a clinical diagnosis and see what kind of brain issues we were dealing with. I made an appointment at the Cleveland Clinic—Lou Ruvo Brain Center, which we are lucky to have in the Las Vegas area—in March 2018. It opened in 2010, the year we had moved to Nevada.

I was stunned by the beauty and significance of the Frank Gehry-designed edifice as we drove up to the building. Built at the corner of an intersection in Symphony Park, it is set apart from other structures. The front of the building is an undulating, chaotic, stainless-steel facade that evokes the complexities and intricacies of the human brain. The entrance at the rear of the building is a no-nonsense clinic structure that inspires confidence, professionalism, and research.

We were greeted by friendly volunteers who led us up the elevator to the quiet waiting room filled with fountains and murals, with scenes evoking tranquility and serenity. It is a peaceful area, and we didn't wait long before being called.

We met with Dr. Adrienne Pan and Dr. Gabriel Leger for the initial assessment, which included a neuropsychic battery of written and oral questions. While I waited, the tests were administered in another room, which took about an hour. When he finished, Mike returned to the examination room, angry and agitated. The test was lengthy and difficult for him. He kept making excuses for his inability to draw a circle, or remember the year or who the president of the United States was. "I get nervous taking these tests and can't remember things," he explained angrily.

"I know," I said, nodding my head. "That's okay. Just keep doing your best."

When I heard the results, I was shocked at how poorly Mike had done on these tests. His performance showed that there was likely an "underlying neurodegenerative process" going on, according to the doctors. They ordered a metabolic PET scan to see areas of damage in the brain and get a diagnosis. Is it Alzheimer's or some other dementia? We scheduled a follow-up visit in July to get the PET scan results.

Four months later, after undergoing the PET scan, we returned to the Cleveland Clinic and sat nervously in the exam room. This was a big moment for both of us. What would the scan of his brain show? When Dr. Marwan Sabbagh entered the room, he smiled. Then he said he could see a buildup of tau proteins in the left posterior temporal lobe and the inferior parietal lobe. This, combined with the oral and written tests Mike had taken, led him to a diagnosis of logopenic progressive aphasia (LPA), a rare dementia that affects language, he told me. It includes language difficulties, due to shrinking or atrophy in those two specific lobes of the brain, as well as memory loss.

Scientists know that with LPA, there is a significant buildup of proteins called amyloid and tau within brain cells, which are the same proteins that build up in Alzheimer's disease. These proteins usually occur, but science does not yet understand why they build up in large amounts in some people. As more and more proteins form, the cells lose their ability to function and eventually die. This causes the affected parts of the brain—most often the left posterior temporal cortex and inferior parietal lobe—to shrink.[1]

Whereas most dementia caused by Alzheimer's disease (60 to 80 percent) starts with memory loss,[2] LPA begins with a loss of language. Dr. Sabbagh said that Mike didn't have Alzheimer's. He had LPA dementia, but Alzheimer's probably caused it. Dementias are the result of damage to different parts of our highly complex brains.

He prescribed 10 mL of memantine twice a day to help slow the decline, and we left feeling that at least we knew a bit about what we were dealing with.

After reading the small pamphlet I was given, I realized I needed more information. I looked up "progression of dementia" on the internet. I discovered that while different kinds of dementia start in various areas of the brain that control various aspects of our behaviors and abilities, as dementia progresses into the middle and later stages, the symptoms of the different dementia types tend to become more similar. This is because more of the brain is affected as dementia progresses.

Over time, regardless of what caused the dementia, the damage spreads, leading to more symptoms because more areas of the brain cannot work

---

1. UCSF Weill Institute for Neurosciences, Memory and Aging Center.

2. World Health Organization.

correctly, nor can they work together. At the same time, already damaged areas become even more affected, causing symptoms the person already has to worsen. Eventually, the disease damages most of the brain. This causes significant changes in all aspects of memory, thinking, language, emotions, behavior, and physical problems.[3] Yikes! I realized that Ratt will continue to gnaw until he damages, disrupts, and kills almost every part of Mike's brain.

When I later read Mike's PET scan report, it indicated that "hypometabolism was more pronounced in the posterior cortical regions. The distribution pattern is consistent with Alzheimer's dementia." *What is hypometabolism,* I wondered? Hypo means lower or below, and metabolism is a group of chemical reactions in the body's cells that create energy. So Mike had low brain energy.

We need this energy to do everything from moving to thinking to growing.[4] Brain metabolism—the engine that powers our thoughts, emotions, and actions—is a delicate balance of energy production and consumption. When this balance is disrupted, the consequences can be profound and far-reaching.[5]

Imagine the brain as a bustling metropolis, with millions of neurons constantly communicating, processing information, and maintaining the myriad functions that keep us alive and thinking. Just like a city needs power to keep its lights on and its systems running, our brains require a constant supply of energy to function optimally. This energy comes primarily from glucose, which is broken down through various metabolic pathways to produce ATP, the cellular energy currency.

---

3. Alzheimer's Society.

4. Britannicakids.com.

5. NeuroLaunch.com. "Where Gray Matter Matters."

Now, picture what would happen if this city suddenly faced an energy crisis. Lights would dim, systems would slow down, and the once-vibrant metropolis would struggle to maintain its normal operations. This is essentially what happens in brain hypometabolism, a state where the brain's energy production and utilization fall below normal levels. It's like a brownout in your neural networks, affecting everything from memory formation to emotional regulation.[6] So Mike's brain was having a brownout. The energy in his brain was dimming and would continue to dim until it was extinguished.

How did Mike, such a bright, engaged, educated man, develop dementia or acquire Alzheimer's if that was indeed the cause, I wondered. If, as his PET scan report indicated, his brain metabolism was consistent with Alzheimer's dementia, did Alzheimer's disease cause his LPA? Harvard.edu states that it is a variant of Alzheimer's. But science does not yet know what causes Alzheimer's.

Mike also had none of the other usual causes of dementia that we were aware of—no weakened blood vessels in the brain, no traumatic brain injury, no infections causing high fever, no metabolic disorders such as thyroid problems or diabetes, no medication issues, vitamin deficiencies, heavy metal or pesticide poisoning, no alcohol abuse, brain tumor or cancer, or a history of smoking. He did not have Parkinson's, Huntington's, or Creutzfeldt–Jakob disease. If Alzheimer's caused his dementia, what caused his Alzheimer's? Why did Ratt enter his brain and begin gnawing away at the neurons?

The doctors at the Cleveland Clinic said they did not know what caused Mike's particular dementia. The overwhelming suspicion was Alzheimer's. But even if they did know, there was no known way to stop

---

6. Mosconi, L. "Glucose Metabolism in Normal Aging and Alzheimer's Disease: Methodological and Physiological Considerations for PET Studies." Clinical and translational imaging. (2013); 1(4), 217–233.

or reverse the progression of any dementia. With the diagnosis, however, I knew now that we had left FrontierWorld and stood firmly in the middle of AdventureWorld. He was in stage 4, early dementia.

The human brain's power, magnitude, and complexity are beyond measure. The brain controls everything that makes us a living human—thought, memory, emotion, awareness, planning, touch, motor skills, vision, breathing, temperature, hunger—every process that regulates our body. The brain is the control center, the black box, that gives us our sense of self and keeps us alive.[7]

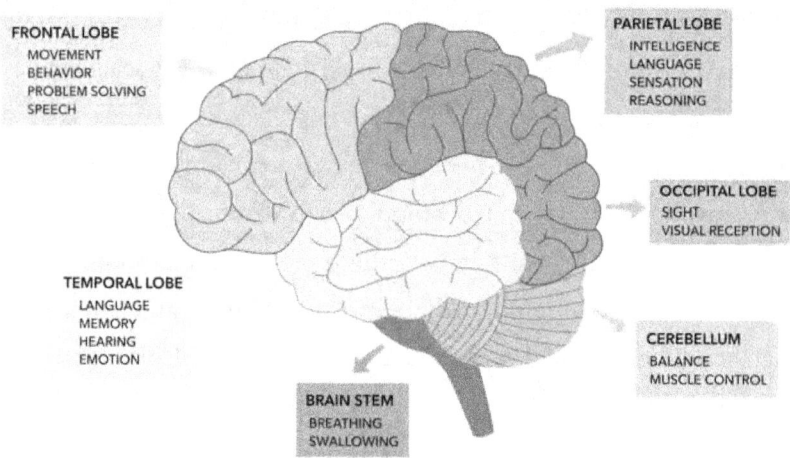

Brain sections and organ part functions.

---

7. Hopkinsmedicine.org.

Intermission

More than eight billion people currently live in Normaland. Fifty-five million souls, like Mike, who used to live there, have tumbled down into the Dementialand pit. This number will almost double every twenty years, reaching 78 million in 2030 and 139 million in 2050.[1] That's a staggering number. Once these poor souls lose their footing, unseen ogres push, pull, and prod them onto an invisible, slippery slide that sweeps them at different speeds down the chute, where they land in a dark and steamy rat hole far below Normaland.

Once humans reach the age of eighty-five, somewhere between 25 and 50 percent of every person alive will fall into Dementialand.[2] That is nearly half of everyone over eighty-five. Reflect on that figure for a minute! If you add in the partners or significant others, the number of people affected by dementia, directly or indirectly, grows exponentially. Dementia is not a normal part of aging. Dementia is brain damage.

Hordes of people have left Normaland and are either sliding into or have arrived in Dementialand, either temporarily as caregivers or loved ones, or permanently as the ones directly affected. Nobody wants to go to this terrible rat's nest. It is the antithesis of Disneyland. Entry tickets result from a randomly cruel lottery of life, with very high odds of winning. And this is one lottery everyone hopes to lose.

---

1. Alzheimer's Disease International.

2. dementiatalkclub.com.

All dementia is progressive, meaning that it will continue to get worse. Think of an imaginary, small rodent trapped in the maze of gray and white matter in the brain, slowly gnawing away at the wiring. As he crawls along, Ratt gobbles up healthy tissue and gradually deprives the person whose body encases the brain of the ability to speak, think, remember, solve problems, and maintain emotional control.

As Ratt moves through the maze of whites and grays, a person in Dementialand may also experience personality changes and behavior problems, such as agitation, delusions, or even hallucinations. Ratt doesn't die; the neurons in the brain do.

Dementia starts slowly as Ratt engages in his carnivorous ravaging. So, while early symptoms differ depending on what part of the brain Ratt attacks first, everyone with dementia ends up the same way. Eventually, Ratt finally reaches the part of the brain that directs eating, swallowing, walking, or breathing, typically eight to ten years after the symptoms begin. With one big chomp, he severs the last remaining nerve fibers. Those functions cease, and life ends ...

What Is Dementia?

It is astounding how many people Mike and I meet who, after observing Mike, are eager to talk about dementia. They mention that they have a parent or grandparent or know someone who has Alzheimer's or dementia. They frequently use the two words interchangeably and usually admit that they don't understand the difference between the two. In the simplest of terms, dementia is brain damage.

Dementia is a catchall–umbrella term that describes brain damage that causes a decline in memory, thinking, language, and social abilities that interferes with everyday activities and relationships. While memory loss is a widespread symptom of dementia, this, by itself, does not mean that a person has moved to Dementialand. If there is significant impairment in two or more brain functions—such as memory and language skills—doctors declare that they have moved to the land beneath Normaland.[3]

Many things besides Alzheimer's can damage the brain. The suspected causes of dementia range from Parkinson's disease to metabolic disorders like thyroid problems or diabetes, brain tumors or cancer, genetics, and damage to blood vessels in the brain. Additionally, traumatic injuries that might be sustained in an accident or repeated brain injury, such as those endured in sports, can cause brain damage. Even some vitamin deficiencies, certain medications, heavy metals, or pesticide poisoning can damage brain cells.

Causes and Types of Dementia

Alzheimer's disease is the most common cause of dementia in the United States. The Alzheimer's Association estimates that this condition affects around 6.7 million people in the US ages sixty-five and older, and almost two-thirds of people are female. A new study about counties in the US where Alzheimer's is more common, lead by Dr. Kumar Rajan, a professor at Rush medical college in Chicago found that "older Black Americans are about twice as likely to get Alzheimer's as white Americans. Hispanic seniors are about 1.5 times as likely to develop it."

But experts don't have the answer yet as to what causes Alzheimer's. They think it's probably due to a combination of natural aging, genetics, things in the environment, and a person's lifestyle, such as what they eat and how much they sleep. Brain imaging scans show the brain changes caused by Alzheimer's. Experts describe them as "plaques and tangles." The first signs are usually memory problems. Some other signs include repeating words or stories, getting lost in familiar places,

---

3. Alzheimer's Association.

forgetting conversations or events, poor judgment, and changes in mood or personality.[4]

Vascular dementia, the second most common type of dementia, occurs when numerous strokes, heart disease, blood clots, or major surgery block the blood flow to the brain. As a result, the individual may develop difficulty understanding concepts, undergo shifts in their emotional and personality traits, and experience memory difficulties. Vascular dementia can occur alongside other types of dementia, leading to a more pronounced decline. While Alzheimer's disease typically starts with memory issues, vascular dementia often begins with difficulty in planning, organizing, and decision-making. Symptoms may include shifts in personality or mood, getting upset easily, poor balance, and an unusual, shuffling walk.

Lewy body dementia is named after the scientist who discovered tiny protein deposits called Lewy bodies that accumulate in the brain, disrupting communication between crucial cells. Although researchers are still working to understand why these proteins clump together, they know that they also appear in other types of dementia. Symptoms of Lewy body dementia include difficulties with clear thinking, decision-making, and focus. Patients may experience visual hallucinations, hear or smell things that aren't real, struggle with language or numbers, become disoriented with time or place, and even experience sleepwalking, talking in their sleep, or trouble walking.

Frontotemporal dementia. The exact cause is still unknown, but it may have a genetic component that includes gene mutations. FTD is a group of brain disorders caused by progressive nerve cell loss in the brain's frontal and temporal lobes, which control behavior, personality, and language. Like other dementias that affect those brain areas, it also

---

4. Webmd.com.

includes abnormal protein accumulations in brain cells, such as tau or TDP-43 proteins. FTD rarely causes memory problems in the early stages. Instead, people exhibit obvious changes in their personality or behavior, a sudden lack of inhibitions in social situations, and challenges in coming up with the right words when speaking or understanding speech. Cell damage occurs in areas of the brain that control planning, judgment, emotions, speech, and movement, such as shakiness, unsteady balance, and muscle spasms.[5][6] As the disease progresses, motor symptoms similar to those seen in Parkinson's disease or amyotrophic lateral sclerosis (ALS) may develop.[7]

Parkinson's disease dementia (PDD). Around half of those living with Parkinson's disease, a neurological condition, experience some degree of cognitive impairment, including changes in memory and thinking abilities. This can get worse over time, making daily life more difficult. Symptoms can begin with short- or long-term memory issues, difficulties getting around places, especially if they're busy or crowded, changes in mood, delusions, or struggles to remember the names of everyday objects.[8]

Logopenic progressive aphasia (LPA), which Mike has, is a very rare form of dementia. It is also a variant of Alzheimer's and a variant of primary progressive aphasia, a type of frontotemporal dementia—a cluster of disorders that results from the degeneration of the frontal or temporal lobes of the brain. It just starts differently from other dementias. These areas include brain tissue involved in speech and language.[9] People affected often have a hard time retaining short-term information and may complain of memory difficulties. As the disease progresses, individuals may lose

---

5. Webmd.com.

6. Mayoclinic.org.

8. Webmd.com.

9. Mayoclinic.org.

speech entirely, and symptoms may become more typical of Alzheimer's disease, such as memory loss and difficulty recognizing familiar faces or finding their way.

Other dementias include Huntington's disease, prion-related dementias like Creutzfeldt–Jakob disease, HIV-associated dementia, and Alcohol-related dementia.

How Is Dementia Diagnosed?

Cognitive tests: These are usually a series of questions, often given by a primary care physician, such as "Do you know what year it is?" and problems to solve, such as "Can you draw a clock showing the current time?" They assess a person's memory, problem-solving, and language skills.

Neurological tests: These assessments involve a physical examination and aim to gauge how well a person's sensory responses, reflexes, and balance skills are functioning.

Brain scans: These show changes in brain structure or obstructions that could cause dementia symptoms. They may include CT, X-ray, MRI, and PET scans.

Cerebrospinal fluid (CSF) tests: A CSF test may help detect some proteins and other dementia-associated components.

Blood tests: Depending on which state a person lives in, their primary care doctor may be able to order a blood test to analyze their beta-amyloid protein levels. These are the proteins associated with Alzheimer's disease. However, this test alone cannot diagnose Alzheimer's and should be combined with a brain scan.[10]

Genetic testing: Some genes can increase a person's risk of dementia. A genetic test reveals if a person with suspected dementia has these genes.

---

10. Medicalnewstoday.com.

Psychiatric evaluation: During this evaluation, a psychiatrist aims to confirm whether dementia may be contributing to changes in a person's behavior. It is not unusual for people to have dementia and depression or another mental health condition at the same time.[11]

How Does Dementia Progress?

Rather than simply using "early-stage," "middle-stage," and "late-stage" dementia as descriptors, the Global Deterioration Scale (GDS) for Assessment of Primary Degenerative Dementia provides a more comprehensive and detailed description. This scale helps better understand the different stages of dementia based on how well a person thinks (their cognitive decline) and functions (their physical abilities).

---

11. Medicalnewstoday.com.

ACT TWO

Dementialand and the Gate to AdventureWorld

Stages 4-7 - Global Deterioration Scale (GDS) / Reisberg Scale

Diagnosis	Stage	Signs and Symptoms	Expected Duration of Stage
Early-stage	Stage 4: Moderate Cognitive Decline	– Difficulty concentrating – Forgets recent events – Cannot manage finances – Cannot travel alone to new places – Difficulty completing tasks – In denial about symptoms – Socialization problems: Withdraws from friends or family – Physician can detect cognitive problems	The average duration of this stage is 2 years.
Mid-stage	Stage 5: Moderately Severe Cognitive Decline	– Major memory deficiencies – Needs assistance with ADLs (dressing, bathing, etc.) – Forgets details like address or phone number – Doesn't know time or date – Doesn't know where they are	The average duration of this stage is 1.5 years.
Mid-stage	Stage 6: Severe Cognitive Decline (Middle Dementia)	– Cannot carry out ADLs without help – Forgets names of family members – Forgets recent events – Forgets major events in past – Difficulty counting down from 10 – Incontinence (loss of bladder control) – Difficulty speaking – Personality and emotional changes – Delusions – Compulsions – Anxiety	The average duration of this stage is 2.5 years.
Late-stage	Stage 7: Severe Cognitive Decline (Middle Dementia)	– Cannot speak or communicate – Require help with most activities – Loss of motor skills – Cannot walk	The average duration of this stage is 1.5 to 2.5 years.

Stages 4-7 Table: Applicable to Scenes 16 through 39

Scene 17

2018: Adventures in AdventureWorld

As devastating as a diagnosis of dementia is, at least we now had a clear picture of what we were dealing with. This was not a temporary condition caused by a lack of some obscure vitamin. This was dementia, and it would gradually get worse.

In April, after Mike's diagnosis, the Grahams had invited us to spend the weekend with them at their home in Fresno, California. Susie was, of course, struggling with MS as well as dementia. Over the years, we had routinely enjoyed playing social bridge whenever we were together. Susie had been a skilled player with a Life Master status in duplicate bridge, but we knew she had quit playing the previous year. Mike and I hadn't played the card game in several years.

As Richard dealt the hands, we sat around the bridge table one evening, chatting and laughing. Mike and Susie followed our lead, gathered their cards, held them, and fanned them out as we had shown them. Then they stared at them blankly. Neither of them seemed to recognize the game nor know what to do next. Richard and I were surprised that neither could sort their hands into suits nor count their high card points, even with our prompting. They were unable to grasp the seemingly simple concept of matching the hearts or spades and arranging them in descending order. The more Richard and I tried to explain, the more confused they became.

It was impossible not to laugh as the scenario resembled an Abbott and Costello "Who's on First" comedy routine. As the futile attempts continued, the four of us were finally convulsed with laughter. Then

Richard, in his calm, never-get-rattled demeanor, suggested that we play "Go Fish" instead of bridge.

"Do you have any fours?" we asked, and they could hunt in their hands and try to find a four. At least they still knew the difference between a four and a queen at that point. With help and gentle encouragement, both Mike and Susie, while not quite mastering the game, managed to play "Go Fish." After several lively games, we folded the deck and watched a movie. Sadly, Susie would succumb to the disease three years later.

After an enjoyable and eye-opening weekend with the Grahams, we drove home. As Mike sat in his easy chair a few evenings later, he pulled me onto his lap, gently kissing my forehead. "I know I'm losing my memory," he whispered tearfully, "but I am happy. I enjoy every day." We hugged and cried softly together for a long time.

I was so emotionally conflicted. I felt so very sad for him. He knew he was declining mentally and that there was nothing he could do about it, and yet, he had somehow come to terms with it. He had made a conscious decision that he could—and would—continue to be happy. If the situation were reversed, I am not sure I could be as optimistic and brave. I bent his head down and kissed him gently on the top of his head.

This bridge episode not only worried me, it also made me curious. I recalled our dinner conversation a decade earlier. Mike had lost his job because he couldn't learn new information about pharmaceutical trials. Yet, playing the game of bridge wasn't new. It was a skill he had learned years ago, but he obviously couldn't remember how to play. I was suddenly interested in the definitions of learning and memory and looked them up.

Learning is the acquisition of skills or knowledge through experience or studying. **Memory** is the ability to remember previous experiences or information acquired through learning. Learning and memory are inextricably linked.[1] In fact, there is no learning without memory. Learning is all about making and strengthening connections between brain cells—neurons. With about 86 billion neurons in the brain, it is estimated that we have about 150 trillion connections, or synapses. This massive network of interconnections gives the brain its immense computational power. Memory must be working for something to be learned.[2] How to play bridge had obviously been acquired, encoded, and stored in his brain many years ago. And while his memory worked, he could recall it. But now, he could no longer retrieve it from the brain vault because this required memory, which he had lost.

I wondered if when Mike was trying to learn new information for his job, was he able to acquire and encode it but not store and recover it? Or was he unable to encode it at all? Either way, had I known earlier that he was having trouble learning, I might have realized that meant he had difficulty with memory. But probably not. I gave it very little thought until years later. I did not associate his admission that he was struggling to learn the pharmaceutical information with memory loss. And since there is no way to cure or slow dementia down, I am not sure that would have made any difference at all.

When I retired on May 1, 2018, I focused on Mike. He was thrilled that I had stopped working. He'd been waiting for me to join the bowling team he and Tom were on, and they held a spot open for me in each league. We could also play more golf, he was delighted to tell me. Between

---

1. Cunnington, Ross. School of Psychology and Queensland Brain Institute, University of Queensland, Australia.

2. American Psychological Association.

those activities, he understood that my long hours at the computer were pursuing my first book, *Bird of Passage*—my memoir—and was very proud of what I was accomplishing. A bird of passage stays in one place for only a short time, moving quickly on to the next. I couldn't think of a better characterization of me and my life. The only exception was that Mike and I had nested thirty years in Southern California, albeit in five homes in four cities.

The two bowling leagues we competed in were senior leagues. They restricted participation to people fifty-five and older, but most bowlers were over seventy. The other rule is that there must also be at least one woman on each team. It was initially surprising to see the number of people over eighty who bowled regularly and a handful who were in their nineties. A couple of people used walkers, and several hurled the ball past the wheels of their wheelchairs. It's an excellent activity for aging adults that promotes physical fitness and mental and emotional well-being through socialization and activity. Judging from these two leagues, it seemed to keep participants active and youthful.

Mike happily drove us as we made the three-mile round trip to the Sunset Hotel and Casino bowling alley twice weekly.

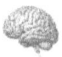

I walked into the hallway Tuesday morning and almost tripped over the double-decker bag that hauls our two bowling balls around. "Why is the bowling bag in the hallway, Michael?" I asked.

"I'm getting ready to put it in the car." Just before we leave for the bowling alley, he positions the ball carrier at the back door so he won't forget it.

"We don't bowl today, my dear. We bowl tomorrow."

"We do? Not today?"

"Nope, tomorrow."

Following me into the living room, he sat in his recliner and shook his head.

"Did we bowl yesterday?" he asked.

"Yes, remember we bowled with Tom and Jo, and Jo went home early with an upset stomach?"

"Wow," he said. "I don't remember that at all."

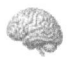

Mike had also forgotten how to do most of the routine household maintenance tasks he'd done automatically only a year ago. The chores that were once shared were now mine alone. I did not need to clutter my brain with that information previously. Now, I found that as Mike had forgotten information, I learned it. I know where the water meter is and how to read it. I know how to set the landscape lighting and the plant watering time. Resetting the various circuit breakers in the main box is a breeze, and I understand why a light socket buzzes and what to do about resetting it. I have set up all the electronics, including Apple Television, the sound bar, the computer, the cable box, and the modem. I also have the phone number of several good handymen for those things I cannot fix, like plumbing or electrical issues.

Knowing that his dementia was progressing, Mike would sometimes look at me, shake his head sadly, and say, "You have to do everything." He knew he could no longer shoulder his share of the household responsibilities, but he was quick to do what he could so as not to feel like a burden.

"Let me put those dishes away. I can do it," he asserted. And indeed, he could. I smiled because I knew that tonight or tomorrow, when I needed to locate a cooking utensil, a particular bowl, or the cutting board, I would begin a hunt like an eager child on Easter morning looking for colorful eggs. He put things in any open space without recognition of order or symmetry. A single glass might end up next to the plates or in with the coffee cups. Finding and rescuing the item later was a minor task, and he felt he was helping. He felt useful. There are several items that I still haven't found, but it will feel like Christmas morning when I do.

"Do you want to set the table for me?" I asked him as I prepared dinner one evening.

"Sure," he agreed happily. "What do you want out?"

"Two forks, two knives, and napkins," I said. This was a task he could perform well only a few weeks ago.

"Like this?" he asked, proudly holding up three spoons and a knife.

"Well, let's use these forks, that knife, and one more knife," I said, taking the spoons and handing him the right utensils. "Now, put out the napkins."

"Where do you keep the napkins?" he asked like a helpful houseguest.

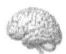

Mike has difficulty following movie plots now, but we binge-watched Breaking Bad in the evenings for the third time, as it was one of his favorites. Because it was familiar, he could follow most of it. He also enjoyed watching football on Sundays and became a fan of the Kansas City Chiefs because he liked the new quarterback, Patrick Mahomes.

Possessing a great sense of humor, Mike always enjoyed a good joke. Yet now, I noticed that when I showed him a particularly funny cartoon in the paper, he didn't understand it. Nor did he understand jokes, puns, or satire any longer. I asked him if he had heard about the two men who stole a calendar. The punch line was that they each got six months. Even though I explained it three different ways, he didn't get it.

Since he could no longer manage websites, I thought it would be helpful if he could Google information he was interested in, so I bought him a senior-friendly, simple smartphone to replace his flip phone. The home page had five big buttons to access—Phone, Contacts, Web, Photos, and Directions. I thought he would be able to use it, but he could not. Was he unable to read the buttons, or did he not understand what the words meant? Whichever it was, he knew immediately that he couldn't learn to use it and insisted I return it. He continued to use the simple flip phone he was familiar with whenever he needed to call me. At least he could still use that … for a while.

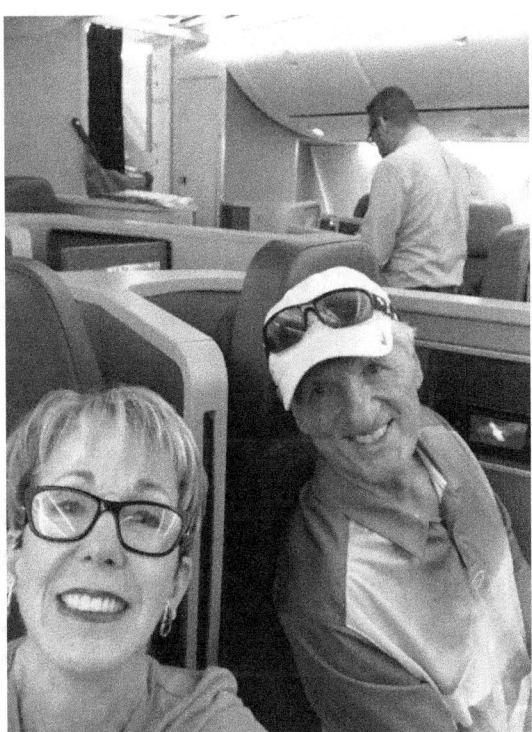

Traveling in comfort to London and Barcelona

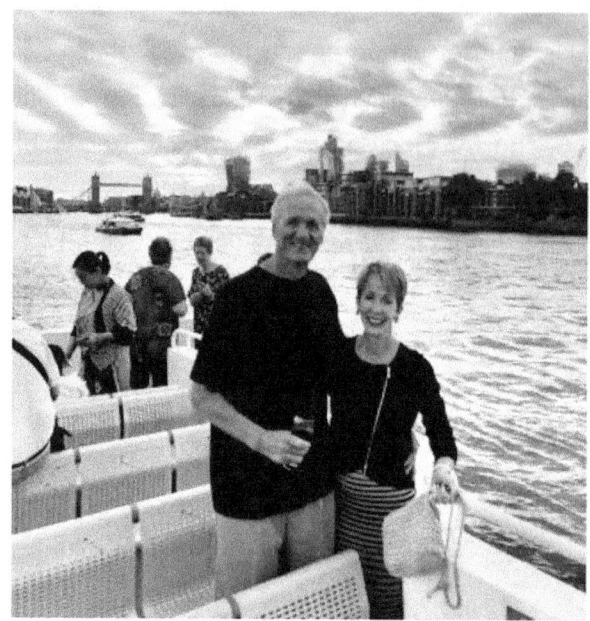

On the River Thames

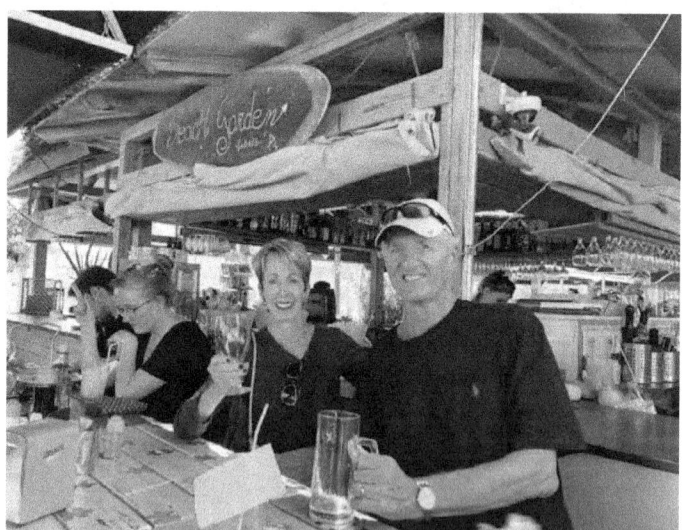

On the beach in Barcelona

Scene 18

Life After the Diagnosis

I often wondered how frequently, if at all, Mike thought about his decline and eventual ending. At some point, would he lose the ability to understand his situation? If so, isn't that at least one good thing about losing one's memory—to forget that you can't remember?

During the summer, we took the grandsons on another European trip. Gavin could not join us this time, so Sunne, Davin, Corben, Mike, and I headed to Paris and Barcelona, two of our favorite cities. Davin, of course, had been to Paris four years before and loved revisiting and showing the others around.

The boys knew about Granddad's recent dementia diagnosis and resulting decline, but Mike still communicated reasonably well. He spoke much less than they were used to, and we needed to watch him closely, as he often became confused about our location and what we were doing. Apart from his inability to speak French or Spanish, he would have had no idea how to find his way back to the hotel if he had separated from us.

One day, Corben recalled, we were sitting at a sidewalk café, and Granddad was evidently trying to ask him about school. "How's the study with the work the ... uh ... books doing?" he asked. That was one of the first times Corben noticed Mike's difficulty retrieving words and composing a coherent sentence.

Mike had been going to a general cardiologist for the last couple of years because of the three ER admissions for rapid heartbeats. He had severe episodes of what he described as electrical currents running throughout his body. After testing, the doctor said that he did not have heart disease or blocked arteries. He did not have Afib. The symptoms that were once dismissed as anxiety attacks turned out to be tachycardia, and there was some damage indicating an earlier silent heart attack. The doctor prescribed the medication metoprolol and asked to see him every three months.

These visits were agonizing to me. They consumed an entire morning or afternoon and didn't eliminate his rapid heartbeats. The good doctor loved to talk about his vast knowledge of the heart. He gave impromptu lectures, complete with diagrams and doodles. He pontificated for forty-five minutes after keeping each patient waiting hours to gain an audience with him.

The wait time is not an exaggeration. It felt as though we were all on an imaginary conveyor belt. After check-in, patients sat in waiting room #1 for a half hour. Then the machinery started up, the belt began to move, and we were deposited into waiting room #2. There, we'd find a half dozen patients who had arrived ahead of us, lounging in chairs, looking tired and dejected, flipping through old magazines or looking at their cell phones.

Apparently, the belt had broken down at this point. Clearing this room could take two hours as the conveyor eventually started up and jerked slowly in fits and starts, moving people out. Finally, with everyone ahead of us gone, someone flipped a switch, and Mike and I began moving again, deposited into a private office where we would await the Grand Poohbah himself. This meant another twenty-to-thirty-minute wait when I would read a book or check my emails. When the good doctor finally entered the office, he would ignore me and greet Mike, asking him how he was doing.

For the first five or six visits, he seemed annoyed that I frequently spoke for Mike. "He has dementia," I reminded him for the third or fourth time, "and it's difficult for him to express himself or understand your questions. So, if I may continue ... he's had several incidents of rapid heartbeats that appear as though he is having a heart attack. They last several minutes, and it's frightening."

"Don't worry, Mrs. Hobbs," he said, finally addressing me. "The only time to be concerned enough to go to the ER is if he passes out." For some reason, this did not seem like sound medical advice to me. Then Dr. Poohbah expounded on various aspects and functions of the heart, pointing at charts and drawings, and declared Mike's heart condition well managed, based on his prescribed medication. He told us to come back in three months and reminded us to go to the ER should he pass out.

Bless Mike's damaged, little brain. He liked him. On the other hand, I thought Dr. Poohbah's arrogance and condescending manner were incredibly annoying, and the time we wasted awaiting his grand entrance irritated me. But I stifled my resentment and tolerated it for two more years because Mike was comfortable with him.

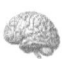

Before the holidays, I posted on FB that we were going to Palm Springs, and since we would be in Southern California, we would love to meet up with available friends. Steve Kenney called and said he and another of Mike's buddies wanted to meet us for lunch one day that week. Since we hadn't spoken since he had let Mike go, I told Steve that Mike had been diagnosed with dementia. They drove from San Diego one morning and met the five of us—Davin, Corben, Sunneshine, Mike, and me—at the designated restaurant.

As we sat on a covered patio of one of our favorite Italian spots, Steve and Terry regaled the assembled group with tales of the incomparable Mike Hobbs. Corben and Davin sat spellbound for the two hours as Mike's friends wove stories of Granddad's years of past triumphs and days of glory, telling inspiring and funny stories. As we hugged goodbye, Steve drew Corben and Davin in and told them how lucky they were to have Mike as a grandfather. The entertaining, lively luncheon and kind parting gesture made a huge impression on both boys and filled my eyes with grateful tears.

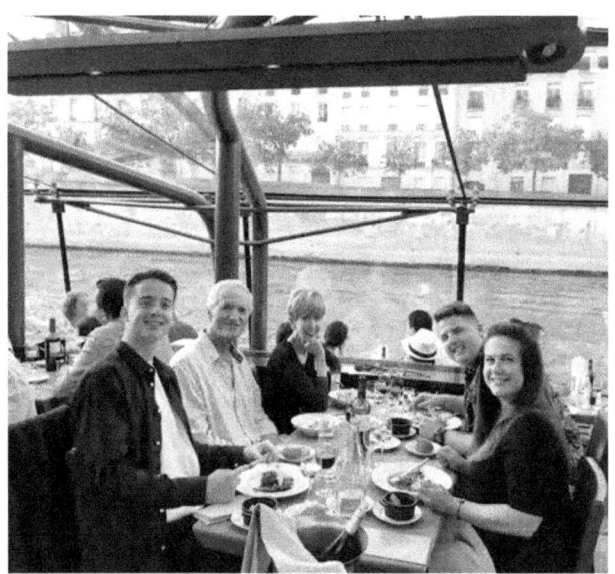

Dinner on the Seine River, Paris

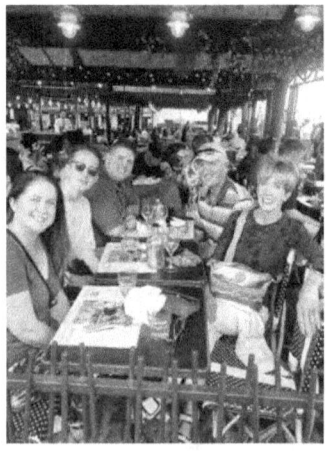

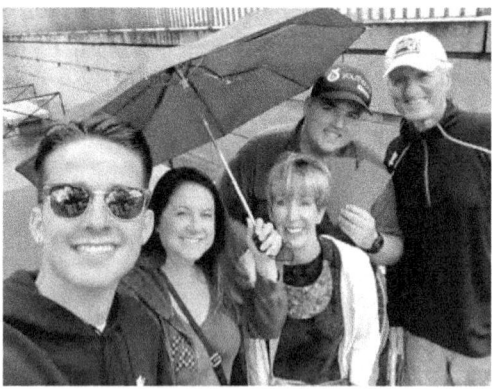

Paris in the rain. From left Corben, Sunne and Davin

Dinner in Montmartre, Paris

Scene 19

2019: One Year After Diagnosis—Memory

Gradually, I took over all the bill-paying, careful not to damage Mike's ego or make him feel brushed aside like so many crumbs on the floor because he had lost the ability to keep track of bills and money. At first, he resisted, insisting on waiting until a bill came in the mail and writing a check to pay it as he had always done. I tried to ease him out by telling him it was better to pay directly from the bank, and we both knew he could not navigate the computer to learn this new skill of online banking. Little by little, it became less and less of an issue as, over the following months, he forgot how or when to pay the bills.

If Mike's failing memory was at the root of most of these issues, where is memory processed, I wondered. What part of what lobe is responsible for memory? Most memory formation happens in the hippocampus, which is in the temporal lobe. However, the process of memory involves not just the hippocampus but many other connected brain regions because there are different kinds of memory. The damage to Mike's left temporal lobe has affected his ability to understand and use language, as well as many aspects of his memory.

Our memory is not just important, it is vital. It helps make us who we are. Without memory, we could not get out of bed in the morning. *Who am I? Where am I? What am I doing?* Our ability to function daily, develop and maintain essential relationships, and recall significant past events relies on memory. Memory is the psychological process of acquiring, storing, keeping, and later retrieving information.[1] Memories are stored like files on a computer that can be accessed whenever needed. They help us form our thoughts and influence how we see the world.[2]

There is not just one part of the brain that controls memory. There are several different kinds of memory for facts, skills, and events in our lives that involve different areas distributed across the brain, each with various processes that rely on other regions. Our brain, therefore, learns by making and strengthening connections between things in memory by association and context. People with damage in particular brain areas have different types of memory loss.[3]

There are three kinds of memory. *Short-term memory* is a temporary storage that holds memories for a few seconds or minutes and is easily accessible. The amount we can keep in our brain at one time is limited, like a phone number or passcode we want to remember for a few minutes to use immediately. *Long-term memory* is like a permanent file that can hold information for years and has unlimited storage. And finally, there is *sensory memory*. That is information collected from our senses: hearing, eyesight, touch, smell, and taste. This is also temporary and is only stored for a few seconds.

To collect and store information for later retrieval—to remember—many parts of the brain must collaborate through neuron pathways, or highways. This is a vital human process for problem-solving or navigating unfamiliar places. It also helps with reasoning and avoiding things that might cause us harm.[4] After falling into a large cactus at three,

---

1. Psychologytoday.com.

2. sciencealert.com. "A Neuroscientist Explains How Your Brain Actually Thinks."

3. solportal.

4. Clevelandclinic.org.

our son, Brett, remembered that cacti needles hurt and didn't have to be told again to avoid them. Memory told him that a cactus is painful.

Human memory involves the ability to save and recover information. However, this process is not flawless. Sometimes, people forget or misremember things, and other times, data is not encoded correctly in the memory bank in the first place.

The information we encode and save into memory does us no good unless we can retrieve it. Our ability to access information enables us to use these memories to make decisions, interact with others, solve problems, and learn. This means that memories must be organized into the brain's filing system in such a way that we can pull them out when needed. "It is as if to make sense of the world, the brain organizes individual, distinct experiences into information clusters or folders so we can access them easier."[5] We have probably all had the experience of forgetting a word or a song and suddenly having it pop into our heads minutes later. It's as though while we have been doing other things, the brain has been quietly searching through its Rolodex filing system to locate and retrieve the forgotten word.

Semantic memory focuses on facts, ideas, and concepts—things we have learned apart from personal experience, such as a history or science lesson. Episodic memory refers to recalling particular and subjective life experiences—biographical experiences the individual has had, like a vacation they took.[6]

Much of Mike's semantic memory has been lost, as evidenced by his inability to learn about pharmaceutical trials. I had hoped he could hold on to some episodic memory for as long as possible. Moreover, I wanted

---

5. sciencedaily.com. Davachi, Lila. NYU Department of Psychology. Senior author of paper appearing in the journal Neuron.

6. Simplypsychology.org.

the boys, his grandsons, to have plenty of their own beautiful episodic memories with Granddad, whom they adored, before Ratt completely destroyed who he once was.

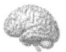

Thinking of episodic memory, I was eager to plan the next journey abroad for Mike and me because next year, on March 28, 2020, Mike and I would celebrate fifty years of marriage, and I wanted to do something special to mark the half century we had officially been together. With his dementia diagnosis, I knew time was running out for him, but I was hoping a trip next year would still be enjoyable and memorable for him.

Enticed by Viking's TV ads, I decided a European river cruise would be an excellent way to celebrate and maybe even renew our vows on board the ship. My sister Cathe, brother-in-law Tom, our cousin Sue, and her husband, Alfred, were enthusiastic when I asked if they would be interested in joining us. So the six of us booked the April 2020 cruise set to sail a week after our fiftieth wedding anniversary—close enough. My plan was for Mike and me to waltz with Strauss as we sailed down the beautiful, blue Danube, celebrating our golden wedding anniversary.

Because we would fly directly to Germany and board a ship that would dock at different cities, this would eliminate having to rush from place to place or tour to tour, which I knew would be difficult and stressful for Mike. We could take the excursions and then reboard the boat. I wouldn't need to schedule hotels or tours. There would be no packing and unpacking. We wouldn't even have to plan meals. No fuss, no muss, I mused. I had plenty of airline points, so I would upgrade to business class so Mike would have a comfortable flight and stretch out his long legs. I knew the trip would be challenging for him, but it would be our last, and we would have family to share the once-in-a-lifetime experience. We had six months to envision, discuss, prime his brain, and wait.

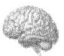

Corben, the youngest grandson, who had always looked up to his grandfather, wanted him to know how much he meant to him while Mike could still understand his words. He sent him a lengthy essay that he had written the year before when he was a sophomore in college, applying for a scholarship. The scholarship committee had assigned a writing prompt: "Who Is Your Role Model, and Why?" Corben had unhesitatingly chosen his grandfather, Mike. In fact, he said, over the years, he had always chosen his grandfather whenever asked to respond to this same query, while most of his colleagues had chosen a celebrity.

When I read his beautiful tribute, it felt like an extraordinary eulogy that most people will never hear about themselves. I read it to Mike several times, and his eyes filled with tears as he realized the impact that he had made on his grandson. Then, as he flipped through the pages, trying to read it himself, overwhelming emotions washed over him as he struggled to locate familiar words. I put the essay in a three-ring notebook, along with pictures of Mike playing basketball and accepting business awards, so he could look at the book and remember some of the things he had accomplished over his lifetime and feel pride in himself. He looked at the notebook daily until, eventually, he reached a point where he could no longer read it, understand its significance, or remember much of his past.

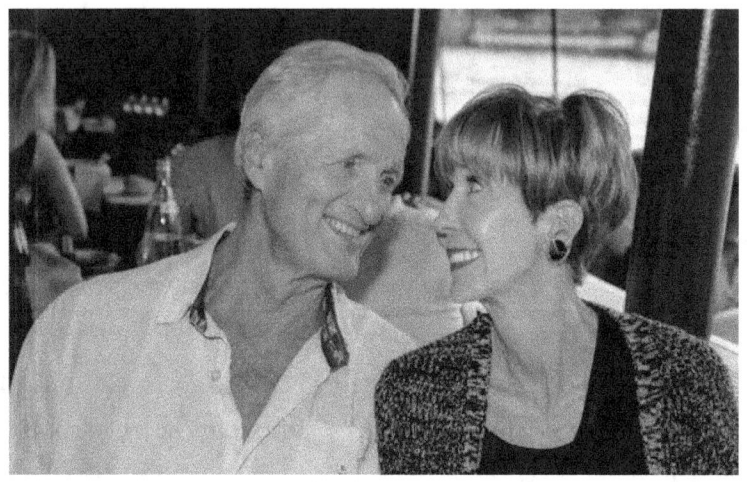

I love you

Scene 20
Mr. Big and the Black Box

In December, we were back at the Cleveland Clinic. It had been six months since Mike's initial diagnosis. This time, we met with a Dr. Miller. Mike was then seventy-one years old. It had been ten years since he lost his job because he couldn't learn new information. The evidence of his dementia had been gradually and slowly progressing. In my mind, the trigger was the untimely and tragic death of our son by suicide on June 6, 2008. When I brought this up, Dr. Miller shook his head. "That's probably not the cause," he said.

Maybe not the cause, I thought, *but surely it could have triggered it or sped up the onset, couldn't it have?* The question plagued me, and Dr. Miller had no answer, at least not one he was comfortable giving me.

Of course, Dr. Miller didn't describe it this way, but his assessment told me we stood firmly in the second park—AdventureWorld—the middle stage. The doctor added 4 mL of Galantamine twice daily to Mike's pillbox, again to slow the decline, and we left, discouraged that not much more could be done.

Over the next few months, we met with more neurologists and clinicians. Each time, they administered different written and verbal tests to chart his regression. "Who is the current vice president? Do you know what year it is? Can you remember these five words and repeat them ten minutes later? Can you draw a clock showing what time it is now? Mike, of course, was trending down in his ability to perform on the tests and continued to protest.

"I do expert sudoku. Tell her, Sherry," he pleaded, pointing at Simrit, the nurse practitioner. "I just get rattled on these tests and can't remember things." It was upsetting, unnerving, and obviously frustrating for him to feel like such a failure after so many years of success.

I told Simrit he was still driving a car near home, with me as a passenger, and paying most of the bills. "And yes, he can still do expert sudoku," I said. She nodded and made a note, apparently not impressed or surprised by this revelation, but advised me to watch him carefully when driving. "It's progressive," she said. *There's that awful word again,* I thought.

I drove home because the trip required the use of freeways, and I mentally reviewed what I had learned. I wanted to understand the changes Mike would experience as Ratt burrowed deeper into his gray matter. Mike's diagnosis included the information that the damage in his brain was specifically in two lobes—the left posterior temporal and the inferior parietal. *What activities are those two lobes in charge of,* I wondered. I needed to know more, so I returned to the computer again to learn about the brain and what each part does.

The human brain is one of the most complex structures in the known universe. The average adult's brain weighs about three pounds. Fat makes up about 60 percent of the brain, with the remaining 40 percent consisting of water, protein, carbohydrates, and salts. The brain itself is not a muscle. It contains blood vessels, nerves, and cells, including neurons and glial cells.[1] Neurons send and receive electrical signals telling the body what to do, think, or feel. Glial cells, often called the "glue" of the nervous system, are non-neuronal cells that do not produce electrical impulses but are cells that support, connect, and protect the neurons. The brain

---

1. hopkinsmedicine.org/health/.

contains billions of these neurons intertwined in intricate networks that are responsible for all of our physiological and cognitive functions.[2]

Jennifer Robinson, a professor of psychology and neuroscience at Auburn University, explains it also using the city–highway analogy. "Imagine your brain as a busy city with lots of streets and buildings. Each part of the brain has a specific job, just like certain areas of a city or certain buildings serve different purposes. When you have a thought, it's like a message traveling through the city, passing from one area to another."

A neuron is a tiny cell that sends and receives signals and messages communicating with other neurons. When you have a thought, neurons in your brain fire up and create electrical impulses. In Dr. Robinson's analogy, these neurons form neural tracts like streets and highways. These impulses tend to travel along similar pathways and release tiny chemicals called neurotransmitters. They are like the construction crew that builds the roads, making delivering messages easier. As we learn, these connections grow stronger.[3]

Damage to the brain, such as that experienced by people with dementia, disrupts communication, causing many neurons to malfunction and eventually die, leading to widespread loss of brain function. Damaged neurons disrupt the neural network, like potholes in a road. Unlike real roads, however, with dementia, these neural potholes cannot be repaired and only grow larger.

The human brain has three major parts: the cerebellum, the brain stem, and the cerebrum. The cerebellum, located at the back of the brain, coordinates movement, balance, and posture. It receives information from the eyes, ears, and nose and helps fine-tune motor activities. Additionally,

---

2. nhnscr.org/blog/left-temporal-lobe-functions-symptoms-and-damage.

3. sciencealert.com. "A Neuroscientist Explains How Your Brain Actually Thinks."

the cerebellum plays a role in learning new motor skills and adapting movements based on sensory input.

The brain stem is located at the bottom of the brain and connects the brain to the spinal cord. It sends messages to the rest of the body to regulate balance, breathing, heart rate, and more.

The cerebrum, where Mike's damage originated, is the largest part of the brain. It is in front and consists of gray matter—the cerebral cortex—and white matter at its center. The cerebrum has tremendous responsibility. It initiates movement, regulates body temperature, and enables speech, judgment, thinking, reasoning, problem-solving, emotions, and learning. For efficiency, the cerebrum delegates this monumental job to four major lobes: the frontal, temporal, parietal, and occipital.[4] Each lobe controls different functions. However, they abut each other and are connected by the neural pathways that allow them to work together to process and share information.[5]

The frontal lobe, located at the front of the brain behind the forehead, is involved in personality characteristics, decision-making, and movement. The prefrontal cortex, located immediately behind the forehead in the frontal lobe, affects behavior, personality, and the ability to plan. It is often called the CEO of the brain—Mr. Big, as I think of it.

The occipital lobe is at the back of the head. It processes what we see with our eyes and records it in memory.

The parietal lobe is between the frontal lobe and the occipital lobe. It helps us identify objects and understand spatial relationships. It processes sensory information from the outside world, mainly relating to spatial sense and navigation. This lobe integrates sensory and motor information, helping us understand our body's position in space. It's critical to finding

---

4. The Cleveland Clinic.

5. kenhub.com/en.library/anatomy/lobes-of-the-brain.

specific locations in our environment and coordinating visual information we see with motor actions we do. It's sort of like an internal GPS.[6]

The temporal lobe is located near the ears on both sides of the brain. It processes information from our senses of smell, taste, and hearing and helps us store memories. This lobe handles auditory perception and is also essential for processing speech and vision—reading.[7]

The left posterior temporal lobe—damaged in Mike's brain—involves higher cognitive functions like learning, problem-solving, and creativity. It plays a critical role in processing language and comprehension, and damage to this lobe unsurprisingly results in language problems. This brain area also processes auditory information, including speech and music. It contributes to our understanding of the meaning of words. It is a type of long-term memory involving the capacity to recall words, concepts, or numbers, which is essential for the use and understanding of language.[8]

The billion-dollar question is: how quickly will the damage increase and expand to other areas of his brain?

---

6. The Cleveland Clinic.

7. sciencenotes.org/parts-of-the-brain-and-their-function.

8. cedars-sinai.org.

Scene 21

2020: Two Years After Diagnosis

In January, just as we were excitedly anticipating our anniversary river cruise on the Danube, now only a couple of months away, a counterpart in China notified HHS Secretary Scott Azar that a "mysterious respiratory illness" was spreading in Wuhan, China. Suddenly, everything changed. It seemed as if the world had stopped revolving and encircling the sun. The United States went into lockdown shortly after that.

The Viking company had no choice but to postpone the trip on the Danube indefinitely. Our golden wedding anniversary on March 28th passed quietly. We were home alone and toasted with a glass of bubbly. We had shared over a half century of life, lessons, and the pursuit of happiness. *"A votre sante,"* I said, smiling. "To your health."

While we waited for the rescheduling of the river cruise, bowling was a big part of our lives. It, too, was stopped for months due to COVID-19, but when it started back up and everyone had been vaccinated, we headed back to the Sunset bowling lanes. Masked like the Dalton gang and avoiding close encounters of any kind, we resumed bowling in both leagues on Mondays and Wednesdays. We played golf frequently with Cathe and Tom, went four-wheeling with the Andrews, and visited the grandsons in Southern California several times. I rented an Aquabike and worked out in our pool. I also bought a cornhole bean bag toss for the backyard that

Mike and I enjoyed in the late afternoon and evenings. Like the rest of the world, COVID kept us cozy.

I worked on my book in between activities, and in September, I published *Bird of Passage*, the memoir I had been writing for the past two years. Mike was thrilled and so proud of me. He paged through it and said that he'd read it, but I don't know how much he could read at that point.

The year 2020 had passed painfully slowly for us, as it did for most people. We kept to ourselves, got vaccinated, wore masks, and mingled mainly with family.

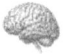

Two years following his diagnosis, Mike was still comfortable driving short distances within a five-mile radius of our house with me in the car. He said that if he got confused about which way to go, he would wait for me to help direct him. His reaction time had slowed, and I took the wheel occasionally, reversing a role we had maintained for over fifty years. Mike had always loved to drive, and, in the past, if the two of us were going anywhere, he wanted to drive, even if it was across the country.

But now, I needed to guide him to most places. I noticed Mike could no longer follow or visualize simple directions requiring him to understand linear information or multiple instructions. If I said, "Go to the end of the street, turn right, then go to the light and make a left," he would shake his head, trying to clear the confusion. His brain could hold only one idea, one instruction at a time. He had lost the ability to picture the directions and visualize the destination. "Okay," I learned to say, "just go to the end of the street. Stop. Now turn right." I motioned with my finger in the right direction because sometimes the words right and left confused him.

New research by neuroscientists at the University of Chicago showed that the posterior parietal cortex—one of the two lobes damaged in Mike's brain—is associated with planning movement and spatial awareness. Spatial navigation is the cognitive ability to determine one's position and plan a route or movement in space. It involves the brain's internal mapping system, essential for daily activities.[1]

Mike became confused about how to get home when he had taken Cathe and Tom to the airport and could not find his way back to me when I had outpatient surgery. Now, he was confused by too many directions because he couldn't picture a map in his head. Sometimes, he'd spin around looking for Bijou, who was at the end of his leash in his hand. The internal GPS in his damaged parietal lobe was malfunctioning.

Mike's speech was becoming increasingly difficult to understand. Many times, he had used the wrong words. "Where's my hat?" he'd say, pointing at his wrist. Thinking of what he wanted to say was sometimes fruitless, and he'd give up. "Never mind. I'll think of it later," he said solemnly. But, of course, he could not. The thought was fleeting and gone forever because he could no longer bring those words out of his cognitive filing cabinet. His ability to remember certain things was limited.

Sometimes, when I spoke to him, he didn't hear me. Partly, it was because of his poor hearing, as he had worn hearing aids for years. But mostly, I think, it was because he took a lot longer to hear and process speech, so I needed to repeat what I was saying several times, slowly. His eyes often looked vacant as he concentrated, trying to understand my words, and his responses were jumbled.

Mike's specific brain damage made it difficult for him not only to communicate with language, but also to remember the names of everyday items and where they were stored. However, at this point, he still remembered to make his bed each morning and how to take care of his personal hygiene, like brushing his teeth and shaving. I laid out his clothes,

---

1. Freedman, David. University of Chicago. .

but he dressed for his daily morning walk with Bijou. She guided him around the neighborhood and to one of two nearby parks and brought him home safely in about forty-five minutes. This allowed me time to read the paper and have my morning coffee, awaiting their return.

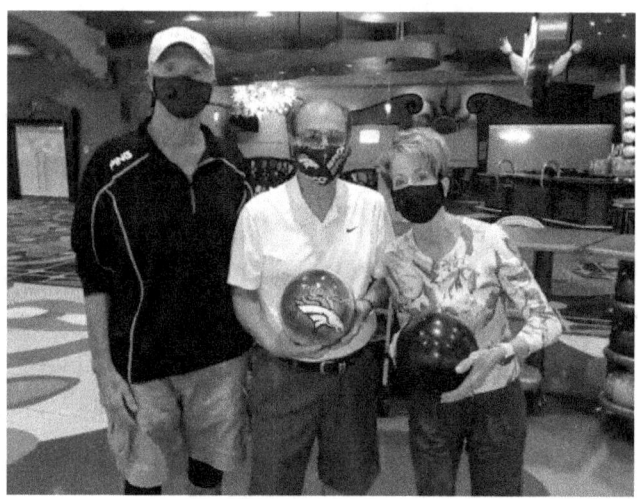

Bowling through Covid with Captain Tom

Scene 22

2021: Three Years After Diagnosis

Instead of listening to the news, which he found challenging and the noise annoying, Mike now watched the news crawl at the bottom of the TV screen. He would pick up something as it scrolled by and try to alert me, but he didn't fully understand it and couldn't explain what he thought he understood.

"Metal flying ground," he said to me one evening at dinner, his eyes wide. I picked up the words and tried to piece the thoughts together.

"A plane?" I asked. "Something about a plane?"

"Yes," he said, nodding vigorously like a small child trying to explain something to their dim-witted parent.

"Are you talking about the engine cover that fell off the United plane with pieces landing on houses in Denver?"

"Yes, yes!" he said excitedly, happy that he was understood.

He could still complete expert-level sudoku, which I found interesting. Clearly, that's a specific compartment of the brain that Ratt had yet to discover. He could somehow pull that stored information out of his memory banks, keeping Ratt at bay by doing it daily.

Mike was bored after he'd walked the dog and finished his morning sudoku. There was not much else he could do. He could no longer write or read and could not follow the intricate dialogue on TV because he didn't understand the words or their meaning. It must be like someone who speaks only English watching TV in his hotel room in Japan. It all must have sounded like gibberish.

I racked my brain, trying to think of tasks that he could do. He folded clothes when I asked him and took the recyclables to the bin when he saw a full container. If I stayed with him, he would mop the floor and run the vacuum for a short time until he lost interest. What else?

"Would you go to the mailbox, honey, and get the mail?"

"Sure," he agreed readily, happy to be of use. "Where are my keys?"

We located the keys, and he went out the front door and walked four houses down to the neighborhood mailbox. "Here's the mail," he said proudly, walking back into the house. "What's this?" He held up the post office key that opened the larger box underneath ours.

"Oh," I said, "we must have a package. I'll walk down and get it." There was no point in explaining what the key was or how to open the larger mailbox. He could no longer recognize or understand what many objects were. And even if he did, he would have forgotten it by the time another mysterious key had appeared in our mailbox.

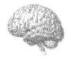

Medically, I was concerned about Mike's heart and tired of feeling manipulated by his cardiologist. After another rapid heart episode, I called a cardio electrophysiologist, Dr. David Navratil, a specialist in electrical cardiac issues, like tachycardia, which Mike had.

After waiting only a few minutes, we were ushered into an exam room, and Dr. Navratil breezed into the room like a whispering wind in a dark, dank forest. Shockingly, there were no interim waiting rooms. He did not even try to impress us with his medical prowess.

After exchanging a few pleasantries, he ran some tests, declared that Mike's heart was healthy, reaffirmed that he did not have Afib, and confirmed the diagnosis of tachycardia, a periodically fast heartbeat over

100 bpm often caused by stress. "I can fix that," he said. "A pacemaker will keep the heart beating regularly."

Whoa! A solution besides going to the ER every few months when his heart raced out of control. We scheduled the procedure, and the doctor implanted a small device in Mike's chest. We visit Dr. Navratil every six months to monitor the pacemaker's battery. He also recorded the heartbeats remotely from a machine next to Mike's chair at home. Since then, Mike has had zero discernible irregular heartbeats, and I have had hours returned to my life.

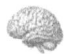

For the first time in fifty years, we began to sleep in separate bedrooms. Mike had decided this abruptly one night, which puzzled me, but as it turned out, it worked well for both of us. He had occasionally lain on his back on the guest room bed, where he claimed the mattress was firmer. Then one day, he decided to sleep there every night. He could fall asleep to the movement of the news on the television a few feet away on the dresser, and I could read myself to sleep in what used to be our bedroom and not worry about disturbing him with a light on. Maybe he moved into that room because he slept on his back like a dead man all night, and I flopped around like a mackerel on a pier. Maybe, when he had the words, he was too nice to say anything and just silently moved into the other bedroom. I will never know what his thought process was.

I worried slightly that we would lose the physical closeness of sharing a bed. But we could still enjoy sex, which became a weekly date in what was now my bedroom. The experience was different, of course. He needed some direction, encouragement, and the help of the blue pill, but he was an eager and loving participant.

He would also occasionally initiate sex after awakening aroused. The blue pill had helped him maintain an erection, but sometime this year, he was no longer able to ejaculate. It was as if Ratt had chewed into the hypothalamus—a gland that controls the hormone system—and snipped the little neurons that talked to the prostate gland, where seminal fluid is stored. The hypothalamus is central to sexual response. This is where sexual stimuli from various parts of the body come together for processing.[1] The brain then sends signals down the spinal cord that cause the body to become aroused and then have an orgasm.[2] In addition, parts of the amygdala in the temporal lobe are crucial in controlling ejaculation.

At first, as one might expect, this inability to have an orgasm was quite frustrating for him. I asked his urologist, who confirmed there was no physical reason causing this. But over the next year, as we continued to have sex, either Mike forgot what he was missing, or he just decided it wasn't going to happen and made the best of it, stopping and showering when he had tired. This went on like this for at least the next three years.

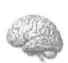

Now, Mike only occasionally wanted to drive us in his truck to the Sunset Station, where we bowled, but it had been several weeks. He usually expected me to drive most of the time. The day was fast approaching when I knew he would be unable to drive at all. He seemed to have accepted that by slowly relinquishing the wheel.

---

1. verywellhealth.com/serotonin-s-role-in-the-biology-of-ejaculation-4156268.

2. Xu Y, X. Zhang, Z. Xiang, et al. "Abnormal functional connectivity between the left medial superior frontal gyrus and amygdala underlying abnormal emotion and premature ejaculation: a resting state fMRI study." *Front Neurosci.* 2021;15:704920.doi:10.3389/fnins.2021.704920.

Fortunately, we never had to have "the talk" about giving up the car keys. A stranger handled it. While stopped at a red light, a woman had rear-ended me. The airbags deployed, preventing any injuries, but the insurance company declared that my twenty-year-old Mercedes Benz was not worth resuscitating and sent me a small check. I put the money down on a 2020 RAV4 Hybrid in March and began driving the new car every time we went out. Mike's eighteen-year-old Ford Expedition sat in the driveway for months. Once a week, I started it to keep the battery charged, but I drove my car everywhere we went. He never asked to drive the RAV4, and I doubted he could learn to use the keyless starter even if he'd wanted to.

Finally, I said, "You know, honey, we need to sell your truck." I girded myself for a tough conversation because I knew he wanted to hold on to the last vestige of his independence.

"It's good to have a backup," he countered.

"Yes, but it's silly to keep paying the insurance, maintenance, and registration fees when we don't drive it."

When he agreed with less resistance than I had feared, I put it up for sale and sold it for thousands less than it was worth to the first person who answered the ad because I wanted to quickly remove it from his sight and mind. Once it was gone, his driving stopped completely.

After that, whenever we drove anywhere, usually to bowling, in typical Mike fashion, he joked he needed a child's steering wheel suctioned to the passenger side dashboard by making steering pantomimes. We laughed at his joke each time we rode in the car, and the joke continued for months.

As we motored along, he looked out the window and chattered, enjoying his new status as a passenger, pointing things out along the way. "Look," he said. "That store is really busy. That's good. It's coming back." He told me about a burning fire in Northern California and that "the bugs (COVID-19) are coming back"—all things he had caught on the news crawl. This told me he could still read some words.

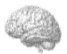

It was a beautiful Saturday afternoon in April. Tom and Cathe picked us up, and we drove to a restaurant in Lake Las Vegas, about twenty minutes from our house, to meet my friend Bobbie Kane. We sat outside on the patio and listened to some beautiful live jazz. Sipping wine and nibbling appetizers, we stayed three hours, entranced and energized by the duo. Mike was usually subdued in social situations now because conversation was very difficult for him to follow. But he laughed and clapped, utterly transfixed by the entertainer. Seeing him come alive—shades of the old Mike—thrilled me.

When we got home, though, he sat in his chair and looked sad. He motioned me to him, and I sat on his lap. "Wasn't that fun?" I asked.

"I can't go anywhere," he whispered. At first, I did not understand what he was trying to tell me. Tom had driven, something Mike would always have done in the past.

"You mean drive somewhere by yourself?" I asked. He nodded. "Does it make you sad?"

"Yes," he replied. "But I still do things myself," he said, looking suddenly hopeful.

"Of course you do. You get dressed yourself and walk the dog. You bowl. You do a lot of things yourself."

"Do they think I'm weak?" I knew he meant declining.

"Do you mean your memory?" He nodded, his head down. "Well, people who knew you before notice a change. You don't talk as much as you used to."

"What do people think of me?" he asked. Then he started to tear up, changing the subject. "I love you so much," he added quickly. "I hope I can be with you forever."

"And you will, my love," I replied. My chest was now heavy, and tears flooded my eyes.

"I talked to people tonight, didn't I?" he asked hopefully.

"Yes, you did," I said. "You laughed and had a great time."

Then he looked at me and said softly, "That was so much fun. I love talking to people."

All I could do was hug him and cry.

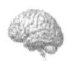

As the months wore on, Mike became increasingly attached to Bijou. "Where's the dog?" he asked frantically, searching under the beds multiple times during the day.

"Honey, she can't go anywhere. She's somewhere in the house or backyard." Eventually, it became such a repetitive question that I began joking, "She took a plane to Detroit." He didn't get the joke, so I eventually quit saying it. But he never stopped asking where she was.

In the summer, he still insisted on walking Bijou every morning, although temperatures were in the nineties and it was quite humid. He reluctantly carried a bottle of water and his phone with him. "I don't need this," he said daily as I slipped the flip phone into his pocket.

"Just take it in case. What if a dog attacked Bijou or you fell down?" I repeated. It didn't occur to me then that perhaps he knew he could no longer use the phone, which was why he knew he didn't need it.

One morning, he did fall, but he and Bijou made it back, only a bit worse for the wear. He stood at the front door and called, "I need help. She pulled me into the mud," he growled, pointing at Bijou, the perpetrator. Dirt and mud caked his right leg and arm.

"Stand there and take off your shorts," I commanded, "and go to the backyard." I hosed him off, removing the layers of dirt. "Now you can go take a shower."

Next, I ran the water over his clothes, shoes, and leash and cleaned his watch. Remarkably, Bijou was unscathed, clean as the proverbial whistle. About an hour later, he looked at me and, apparently having forgotten about the incident, said brightly, "We had a good walk today. It wasn't as hot."

"Good walk?" I said with a skeptical look on my face. "You fell in the mud."

He stared at me for a few seconds, apparently remembering, then said, "Well, I got up."

"That you did." I laughed, and he chuckled right along with me.

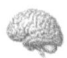

I knew Mike's ability to navigate his environment had deteriorated, and his internal GPS was not functioning well. Even at the bowling alley, he would quickly become disoriented if he lost sight of me when standing only a few steps away. However, I did not expect him to get so confused riding in a car on a trip we had taken countless times.

By my calculation, with the benefit of hindsight, it had been thirteen years since we stumbled into Dementialand and three years since the diagnosis. Mike had grown comfortable in our Henderson house with its predictable surroundings. Even at home, though, he had difficulty finding the garage or kitchen when I asked him to go there. I wasn't sure if it was the spatial relations piece or if he just didn't recognize the word for garage, kitchen, or some combination of both.

We hadn't driven to California in a year. Of course, I didn't know the impact that taking him out of his comfort zone with a malfunctioning internal GPS would have until we left it, but I was about to find out.

We drove to California to see Corben, our youngest grandson, and his girlfriend, Lauryn, graduate from California State University-San Marcos. During the five-hour drive, Mike kept asking where we were going and why, and of course, I repeatedly told him. He also kept asking about Bijou, who stayed with Cathe and Tom.

His confusion about the drive to California—something we had done many times—surprised me. But the environment he was familiar with in his current state had suddenly changed, and he couldn't orient himself to a moving location. We were in my car, but we were not going to the bowling alley. *Where am I? Where am I going? Where is my dog?* he must have thought. I saw a kind of panic set in, as if he feared being kidnapped and secreted away from his safe place.

Five hours after we had left Henderson, we pulled up in front of the Marriott Courtyard in Temecula. I parked the car and stepped out, stretching my back. Mike opened his door and stood staring at the unfamiliar building with a look of abject horror on his face. With his mouth wide open, he stared at the hotel, then back at me, then back at the hotel, then back at me.

"What are you *doing?*" he cried, emphasizing the last word. He looked so terrified, I almost expected the next words out of his mouth to be, "Put the gun down, Sherry!"

I was shocked. *Did he think I was dropping him off at a nursing home?* Why was he reacting this way? I explained again that we were at a hotel in California to see our grandson Corben graduate from college. It had never occurred to me that he would not understand that we were nowhere near home and were in another state. After all, we had lived in California for thirty years and traveled back and forth frequently. But his brain could not make the connection.

After a few minutes, he appeared to have calmed down, and I led him into the hotel, where I checked in. I had planned for Corben, Lauryn, Davin, and Sunne to meet us at the hotel to toast the big event and open gifts before we all went to dinner. The ceremony would take place the next day.

Mike and I took the suitcases up to the room and returned to the lobby where the group was waiting. Mike still seemed slightly suspicious but less anxious. I had taken him away from home, and it was obviously terrifying. Just as he had felt isolated in France when Davin and I left him alone in his room nursing a cold, he could no longer speak the language here in the US, and I was not sure he could use his phone to call me anymore, either. It must be disorienting and frightening to be in a strange place, fearing that you could be left alone with strangers and not know how to return to your safe place.

We located a cozy, couch-filled area and sat around a coffee table. After hugs all around, I popped the cork on a champagne bottle I had brought for the occasion. We munched hors d'oeuvres and chatted excitedly, and the two soon-to-be graduates opened their graduation gifts. Mike seemed to relax a bit as he recognized the group and saw the expressions of love and joy on everyone's faces. That night in the room, though, he had difficulty understanding where we were and where everything in the bathroom was located. This was not his familiar home. I began to have trepidations about our upcoming, yet-to-be-rescheduled Viking trip on the Danube.

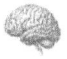

At long last, the big excursion I'd planned two years earlier looked as though it might soon become a reality. I had booked this cruise in 2019 for April 2020, scheduling it for a week after our fiftieth wedding anniversary, with plans to renew our vows on board the ship. "COVID killed the carefully concocted cruise," I said, chuckling, enjoying my alliteration even if he couldn't appreciate it. This was to be our last European trip, and I knew it would have been challenging for Mike even if we had been able to go in 2020. It was now over a year and a half later. Much had changed with Mike's dementia.

It had, of course, advanced. It was a battle of wills between Ratt and me. I knew I couldn't defeat Ratt, but could I wound him with my imaginary saber and slow him down? I was determined that Mike would be able to enjoy the trip and remember it for a while with the help of photos.

Based on the experience during the brief trip to California, it was apparent that Mike's ability to cope with a change in surroundings was in doubt. And flying to Europe and staying aboard a ship was indeed a big change from his usual milieu. Every day, I talked to him about the incredible voyage we would be going on. I showed him the brochures and tried to keep his focus on the future trip.

At last, in September 2021, we got word that the river cruise would finally take place the following month, the second week of October. Of course, everyone, including the crew and staff, had to be fully vaccinated, but the ship would sail. I felt elated because I had feared another delay would be too late for Mike. He was anxious about leaving Bijou and increasingly uncomfortable with strange surroundings and people he didn't know. I assured him that my brother would take loving care of Bijou, which seemed to appease him, although I had to continually reassure him. The fact that my sister and brother-in-law would be on the trip also appeared to have calmed his anxieties, but I don't think he was sure where we were going, why, or when.

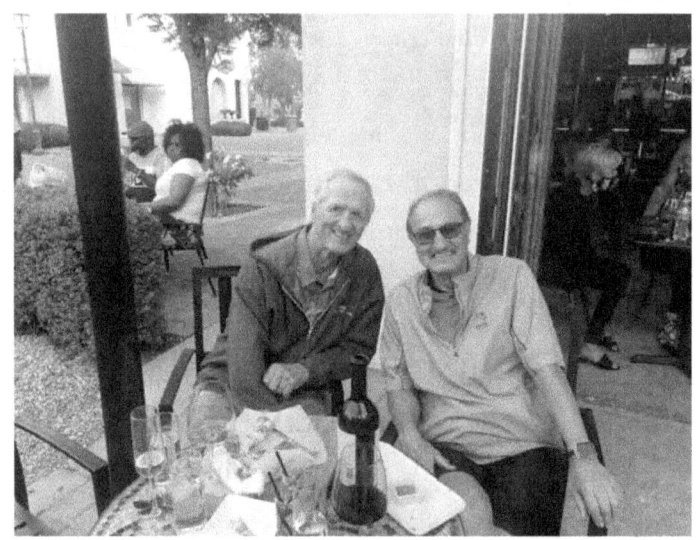

Mike enjoying jazz with Tom

Scene 23

AdventureWorld on the Danube

Stage 5 - Global Deterioration Scale (GDS) / Reisberg Scale			
Diagnosis	Stage	Signs and Symptoms	Expected Duration of Stage
Mid-stage	Stage 5: Moderately Severe Cognitive Decline	– Major memory deficiencies – Needs assistance with ADLs (dressing, bathing, etc.) – Forgets details like address or phone number – Doesn't know time or date – Doesn't know where they are	The average duration of this stage is 1.5 years.

Stage 5 Table: Applicable to Scenes 23 through 33

Our cousin Sue and her husband, Alfred, drove here from Southern California the day before our flight, and the six of us Ubered to the airport together. There, we began the onerous process of checking in with passports and COVID-19 vaccination cards—which needed to be uploaded online at a kiosk—checking bags, etc. We had Global Entry cards to speed us through TSA and customs. Everything was a flurry of confusion for Mike, who stood close to me and looked around as if he had never been in an airport before.

After a long flight out of Dallas, with upgraded business-class seats where Mike could stretch out, sleep, and pat my arm frequently, we had arrived in Munich, Germany. Viking staff met us and a few fellow passengers near the baggage claim area at the passenger pickup. They assisted and led us to a coach for a two-hour ride to Regensburg, where the ship was docked, and there, we boarded the beautiful Viking Jarl moored on the Danube. The weather was like a perfect fall day in San Diego—in the seventies.

We checked into our cabin immediately, and I unpacked and put everything away in closets and cupboards. Although smaller than a standard hotel room, the staterooms were lovely, and the bathroom and shower area was quite roomy. I had upgraded to a balcony, as I had envisioned sitting in the evening with a glass of wine while we motored past charming European villages.

Cocktail hour was every afternoon at 5:30, and I held Mike's hand as we made our way upstairs to meet the group in the palatial bar and cocktail lounge shortly after getting settled in our room. We were excitedly chatting and taking in the festive environment when the program director began her welcome speech and details of the upcoming events. This included information that a daily COVID test for every passenger would be required. We would each spit into a vial that we were to leave outside our door, to be collected each morning before breakfast.

Suddenly, in the midst of the presentation, Mike became uncharacteristically furious. "What are they trying to do?" he roared. "I will not sit here and listen to this." Then he stood up. The room fell into a hush, and everyone turned toward us. I stared, my jaw dropping and mouth forming a large, lipsticked capital O.

"What are you angry about, honey?" I finally asked, shocked at this abrupt and inexplicable reaction. "Do you want to leave? Let's go." He looked around, confused, and then, apparently realizing that his emotion was not the norm, sat back with an angry look and stayed for the duration of the welcome speech.

Dinner followed at seven downstairs in the dining room. It was a sumptuous meal with various appetizers, entrées, salads, and dessert choices. All of us were having a good time, and Mike appeared to have relaxed and enjoyed the evening. I breathed a small sigh of relief.

Tired from the long flights, we all turned in early, skipping the music and dancing in the lounge. We were excited about taking a tour of Regensburg in the morning before we sailed, so we headed up to our rooms for a much-needed good night's sleep.

It took Mike a long time to understand that Bijou was not in the room and would not be joining us. He really could not comprehend where we were or why. I guided him around the small bathroom as he brushed his teeth and got ready for bed.

That night, ensconced in our cabin, he said that he felt as though he had to urinate frequently but could not. "It hurts," he said to me. "I just have to try again." This went on all night, every ten or fifteen minutes. And because the room was unfamiliar, he could not find the bathroom.

The door to the hallway had a full-length mirror hanging on it, and every time he got out of bed to go to the bathroom, he would see the reflection of the bed behind him and become even more confused and disoriented. He walked into the hall in his underwear twice, looking for the bathroom door. Even when I had left it open with the light on, he failed to recognize it. So, every ten or fifteen minutes, I would get up, guide him to the bathroom, wait while he tried again to urinate, and lead him back to bed like a good seeing-eye dog.

As I reflect on it today, it may partly have been the mirror confusing him. If I had thought about covering it, he might have been able to navigate the ten steps. But I was too tired to think straight, and neither of us got any sleep that first night.

In the morning, still in Regensburg, I suspected he had a urinary tract infection. I spoke with Harry, the manager on board, and inquired about a doctor in town. He told me that the fastest and most efficient way to get urgent medical help would be to take a cab to the hospital and visit the ER, which we did. The rest of the group toured Regensburg while we toured the hospital ER.

The European healthcare system worked quickly and efficiently. They immediately took us into an examination room, where they poked, prodded, and peered at Mike. While we waited, the young doctors huddled, took blood and urine samples, and processed all the lab work right there in the ER.

When the lab report came back, the absence of infection in the urine sample surprised me. The young female doctor who had attended to us told me that since he did not have an infection and was not currently experiencing any pain, he had likely passed a kidney stone. She did an ultrasound to see if any additional stones were lurking in his urinary tract.

Following the ultrasound, she pulled her stool up to me and said that while she saw no more stones, she did see some things that concerned her. Along with the observation of unidentifiable spots on his liver, she noted an enlargement in his prostate. She urged me to follow up with a urologist. No need to rush, though, she said when I told her we were on a river cruise. A week would make no difference if he were out of pain. I decided we should split the difference. We would stay the rest of the week enjoying part of our long-anticipated trip and cancel the three-day extension in Budapest. Six more days would be plenty under the circumstances, I reasoned.

When we left the ship that morning to take a cab to the ER, Stojan, who manned the Viking reception desk, had given me a card with locations and two times on it—12:30 and 4:30—where we could take a taxi and meet up with Sabine, the entertainment/tour guide. He explained that those were the meeting places for people on various tours to catch the van back to the boat. I assumed that was what we needed to do to join a tour. "If we are between those times, can we just return to the boat?" I asked him.

"Yes, yes," he replied, giving me a card with the ship's dock number printed on it. However, he forgot to add one tiny yet very important piece of information—the ship was leaving shortly and would not be in Regensburg.

We left the hospital at noon, and, not in the mood to join a tour, I decided to take a cab back to the ship. I handed the driver the card with the dock number on it, and he took us to the indicated spot. Imagine my surprise when we stared at the empty slip. "Where's the ship?" I asked the cab driver.

"I don't know," he replied. "That's the slip number on the card."

But the ship was not there. *Poof!* Gone. It had vanished like a coin in a magician's hand. Apparently, lost in translation was the fact that we were supposed to meet Sabine at those exact times because the boat left shortly after we did, and the tour vans drove on to the next port to meet the Jarl, in this case, now in Passau, Germany. After calling Sabine and explaining our dilemma, she redirected the tour van and returned to the former slip to retrieve us, taking us to the boat in Passau. Like shipwrecked sailors, our crew rescued and reunited us with our fellow travelers.

That afternoon, I emailed our travel agent to request that she kindly cancel the extended Budapest portion of the trip. I explained that we needed to get home and see a urologist. Fortunately, we had purchased insurance for trip disruption, for which his medical emergency certainly qualified. The travel agent rescheduled the flights, and I looked forward to day two of the long-awaited and recently feared five days to follow.

Mike seemed to feel better and out of pain that afternoon. That night, the second night of our trip, we had met the group for cocktails and regaled each other with our diverse and eventful day. Our off-the-grid itinerary won the prize for being the most unexpected and unusual. The others had skipped the available tours, walked around the small Regensburg central square by the boat, and declared that we had missed little—mostly gift shops and curio boutiques.

I breathed a sigh of relief, feeling as if Mike and I might be able to tour Passau in the morning, enjoy the next few days, and then motor on to Vienna and then Budapest, where we were now booked to fly home. We headed to the dining room, relaxed and ready to enjoy the trip. The restaurant service staff was incredibly entertaining and gregarious. Pol and Jay, a young comedy–waitstaff team, remembered each of our names and attended to our every need, want, or wish ... gastronomically speaking.

Tired from the sleepless night before and a most eventful day, Mike and I headed up to our cabin soon after dinner and fell into a deep, much-needed sleep, like two bears readying for hibernation. At about 2:00 a.m., Mike awoke and experienced the frequent need to urinate once again, with a repeat of the previous night with me guiding him back and forth to the restroom. Again, sleep was, at best, intermittent.

The next day, making frequent restroom stops, Mike and I took a brief tour of Passau, fully armed with umbrellas to protect us from the light drizzle and masks to shield us from COVID-19. Because of his dementia and inability to explain what he was experiencing, I did not understand that these frequent bathroom stops were still not productive. Urine was building up in his bladder, filling like a giant water balloon, and he could not release it.

That night, Wednesday, he awoke again at 2:00 a.m., screaming in such pain that I was frantic. He cried and begged me to help him, not understanding that I had no way to summon a doctor. "We were in the middle of a river somewhere between Passau, Germany, and Vienna, Austria. No doctor was on board, and it was now three o'clock in the morning.

"The pain. It's like a hammer hitting me on my back!" he screamed. I have never felt so helpless in my life. Here was a problem that I couldn't fix. When Mike finally yelled again that the pain was in his lower back, I remembered I had packed pain pills prescribed for his chronic arthritic back before we left and gave him two 100 mg pain pills. Magically, the excruciating pain subsided in twenty minutes. I did not associate the pain in his back at that moment with pain in his kidneys, but that's what it was. We finally slept for a few more hours.

The following day, I spoke again with Harry, the manager. "Is there an ER in Krems, Austria, where we will port briefly?" I inquired.

"Yes, yes, there certainly is, but if you were to get off the boat, which will only be in port for a short time, you would miss it and need to take a train to Vienna to fly home. You'd be better off waiting until we arrive in Vienna this evening at seven o'clock. I will arrange to have a doctor board the ship as soon as we dock." I sighed with great relief and thanked him.

Mike and I joined the others at our chosen table for dinner, and he ate very little, spending most of the time in the bathroom.

We docked in Vienna at 7 p.m. and ate dinner while awaiting the doctor. At 8 p.m., Stephan notified me that the doctor had arrived. He was a handsome, young man in his late twenties, probably a medical student or intern, I guessed. He asked Mike to lie down on his back on the bed and felt his abdomen. A senior doctor, who had waited outside in a car, came in briefly to examine Mike and confirm the younger man's diagnosis. The doctor said that Mike could not urinate because something was blocking his urethra. He told me that his bladder was full and he needed to have it drained and catheterized, so he called for an ambulance.

With sirens blaring and lights flashing, the ambulance had arrived. Naturally, with all this excitement, many other passengers came to watch the proceedings as if this was one of the scheduled tours. Against protocol, due to his dementia, they allowed me to ride in the back of the ambulance, and I held Mike's hand as we made our way to the hospital. The poor guy was so confused at this point, with no idea what was happening, where he was, or where we were going. For me, it was just another ride in AdventureWorld. We ended up in our second ER, this time in Vienna. *What an unusual way to see foreign countries*, I thought.

At the hospital, they drained Mike's bladder and fitted him with a colossal catheter about the size of a microwave oven. Then we took a cab back to the ship with the bag hanging on his waist, filling up with the bright-yellow liquid. This was not the vacation I had, of course, anticipated for two years, but he was out of pain and did not have to urinate. I silently thanked the bladder gods.

On day three, we took a brief tour of Vienna with this monstrosity of a bag half-filled with urine hanging from his waist. It was hot, and there was no adequate way to disguise it. We must have looked like unusual tourists, but no one appeared to give us a second glance. I am sure many people were later punching their cell phones, exclaiming, "Wait until I tell you about these crazy Americans I saw today!" Fortunately, Mike was clueless about how he looked. All he knew was that he was comfortable for the first time in several days, and he smiled and thoroughly enjoyed the pain-free tour.

That afternoon, I'd spent three hours on the phone with British Airways trying to rebook flights to go home immediately out of Vienna, not in four days when we reached Budapest. The travel agent could not help me because I had booked the flights separately, wanting to use points to upgrade the seats to business class. I told them Mike urgently needed to see a urologist, that he was wearing a bag of urine the size of a small child, and that I did not see myself spending our vacation draining his urine bag periodically as we toured the landmarks, or leading Mike around with a large bag of pee strapped to his leg. And most importantly, we needed to find out what was causing the blockage.

British Airways was very uncooperative. I explained the emergency and that we had to get home quickly. The first person I spoke with insisted that since we had booked business-class seats, we would, by God, return in business-class seats, even if it meant waiting a week because there were none available. I had told them I didn't care about business class at this point. We needed to leave the next day, as the ship would move on, and the primary airport in Vienna would be in our rearview mirror.

The agent was intransigent. Rules were rules. Customer service and emergencies be damned. When I was on the verge of tears, hysteria, and an anxiety attack, I had begun looking for a hotel in Vienna to wait for the first available flight. Finally, I called British Airways back and found a kind soul who had arranged business-class flights for the following day. We packed and bid a fond farewell to the group.

So long, fabulous river cruise, I thought. *It was indeed a real adventure.*

When we had arrived at the airport, I positioned Mike and his large, rubber appendage in a wheelchair. With the savvy assistance of airport staff, they whisked us through customs, security, and airport terminals. I tipped them generously as we would have never made the flight without their efficiency and knowledge of the airport's hidden passageways.

Once home, we met with a urologist. After testing, he recommended an operation called a Urolift. At the end of December, Mike had the operation. This essentially lifts and secures the enlarged prostate—which the doctor in Regensburg had seen on the ultrasound—off and away from the urethra. This was the culprit blocking his ability to urinate, not kidney stones. I spent the night in a chair by Mike's hospital bed because, of course, he had no idea where he was or why he was there. But the flow could go.

Mike had to continue wearing a catheter, albeit a much smaller one, for months until he could urinate on his own. This was not an enjoyable time for either of us as he was, of course, unable to attend to emptying his bag of pee-pee, which needed to be drained several times a day by yours truly.

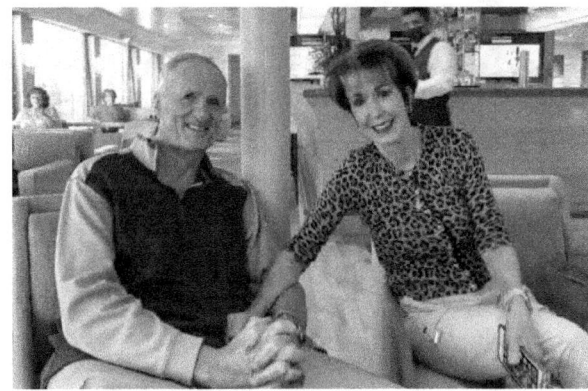

Day one. High expectations for a great trip

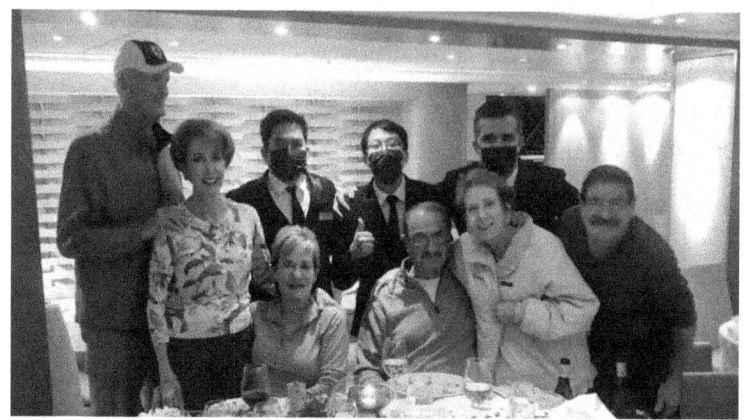

First night with Tom, Cathe, Sue and Alfred

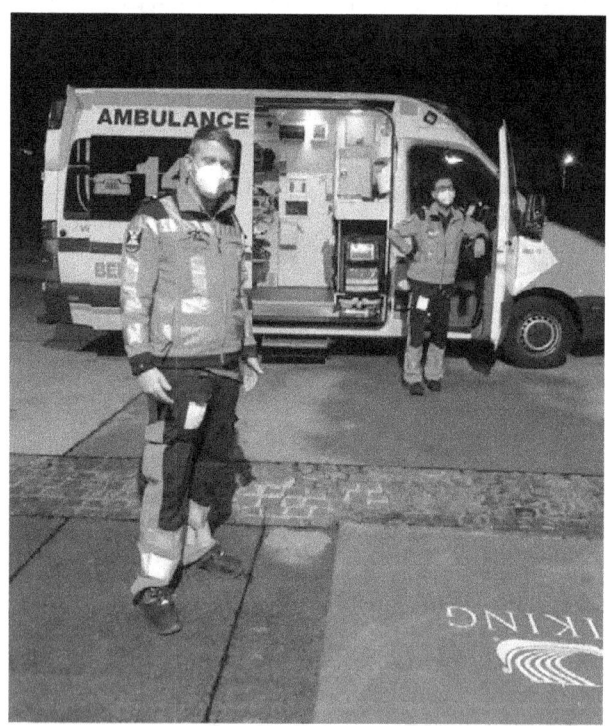

Off to the Vienna ER from the Viking Jarl

Scene 24

2022: Four Years After Diagnosis

For the first few months of the year, Mike continued to walk the dog by himself without being bothered by the smaller urinary drainage bag. Although the temperatures were in the forties, he refused to wear his heavy coat, preferring layers of clothing, and reluctantly took his phone and a bottle of water on the walk because I insisted and persisted. After the operation, we had to suspend bowling for a time, but he was healing and content.

By summer, Mike's morning routine had changed very little, except that he was no longer plagued with a urinary issue. The Urolift had worked as advertised. He still dressed himself to take the dog for a walk, needing no help from me. He referred to Bijou now as he and him. Although I doubted she would have requested those pronouns, she didn't seem to mind.

When they returned, he washed and dried his sweaty clothes—it was summer—and then lay back on the bed, relaxing his back. Every day after walking the dog, he said the same thing, "I'm the only one." He clearly thought about the fact that he seldom encountered others walking their dogs at the same time. However, he could not reason or understand plausible explanations as to why others might not be out walking, nor did he seem to want any.

"They usually go out earlier, before they go to work," I offered initially, but it was as if I had said, "Bandersnatch." It had no meaning or relevance

to him, and he repeated his declaration daily, like a mantra. I quit trying
to offer reasons and just agreed with him.

At this point, Mike still remembered to take his medications, which
I left in the container by his bed. He also made his lunch each day
at noon. It was the same thing—a peanut butter and jelly sandwich,
a handful of raisins, three chocolate chip cookies, and a Diet Coke.
He usually lay on the bed in the afternoon to stretch his back, but
sometimes, he got into the pool and floated on the raft.

Communications were short. "How are you feeling?"

"Good."

He asked me about the temperature, bowling, and the day of the
week. He remembered that we bowled every Monday and Wednesday,
which was the highlight of his week. He lived for bowling and still had
a good solid 150 bowling average.

On Sundays, we usually went out to dinner to get Mexican food. I
had Bijou certified as a "therapy dog," and the company sent her a nifty
harness that warned off petting and let her into restaurants. Naturally,
we took Bijou to Chavelos, and she sat quietly on the bench next to
one of us, looking out as customers came and went. Mike could no
longer read menus, so he relied on me to select his entrée, which I
alternated between chicken burritos and chicken quesadillas. He also
enjoyed chips and bean dip and a glass of red wine.

Having fully recovered from the urological surgery, Mike was
physically healthy. He took no medications, except for the two brain
enhancers and metoprolol for his tachycardia. He regularly asked me
to confirm that he was medically healthy. "My heart is great, isn't it?
My doctor ... what's his name? He is great, isn't he? My dad lived a long
time, to eighty-four, and he was a heavy smoker." These words seemed
to come quickly and easily in rapid fire.

"Yes," I assured him. "You are in great shape."

Mike was happiest when we were about to bowl. In fact, he was giddy. All the way there, he laughed and joked about killing the opponents. "Gonna win money. Get points," he'd said repeatedly. On Wednesday, as we were about to leave the house to drive to Sunset Station, Mike bent down to pet Bijou and offered reassurance. "Don't worry," he said. "We'll be back in two years." It's a good thing Bijou doesn't understand language, either.

In a moment of clarity and nostalgia one evening, Mike looked through the memory books—pictures from our past vacations—and mentioned that he would like to see Paris again. He wanted to revisit a place that he still had some memories of, but of course, he did not know what getting there would entail or how he would feel once so far away from home. It was just a fleeting thought. I should probably have just let it go. He would have forgotten shortly.

But I was grasping at straws, desperate for one last trip to Europe that we could savor and enjoy. The one on the Danube had been a disaster, cut short because of his medical issues, so I decided, on the spur of the moment, that I should book a river cruise up the Seine from Paris to Normandy. He loved Paris, and the ship would take us back to the historic WWII landing in Normandy, which he revered. I received a partial refund for the Danube trip, and I immediately called the travel agent and booked a Viking River Cruise on the Seine for August. I focused on his good physical health and suppressed the part about his memory, inability to understand language, and malfunctioning internal GPS.

In retrospect, this was a fool's errand he had unwittingly sent me on, and I raced to accomplish this as time in his memory hourglass was running out. I knew full well that every day was one more day Mike could decline mentally. Frankly, it was probably a bit selfish. I wanted us to go back and experience Paris so badly that I blocked out his obvious inability to fully enjoy it. I was willing him to feel the same excitement that I felt, but he was incapable.

The original Danube trip planned for July 2020 before COVID-19 derailed it would have been pushing it for Mike's ability to enjoy and fully participate. But certainly, too much had changed in the ensuing two and a half years to expect a relaxing trip motoring down the Seine River where we could chat, sip wine, and share the day's events. I can see now that I was looking through my rose-colored sunglasses, wearing blinders.

I called Cathe and Tom. They weren't ready to take another trip. They, after all, had a wonderful Danube cruise and an extra few days in Budapest. Sue and Alfred had a conflict with the dates, and I didn't want to push the dates out any farther because of the likelihood of his decline. Mike and I would be on our own. This reality hadn't hit me yet. I pressed forward. Once again, I booked our flights to use points to upgrade to business class, crossed my fingers, and then bit my nails down to the quick. July was only two months away.

By fall, I had finished writing my second book, *Mac: The Wind Beneath My Wings*, and needed a new project. I have a bit of an artistic flair, so I'd decided to paint flowers on the stuccoed walls of our garden. Pleased with the result, I then moved inside, painting various floral arrangements and still lifes on different walls inside the house, where the stark blankness called to me. Mike, who would have had a coronary if I had attempted to "deface" the walls only five years earlier, watched blankly as I painted colorful designs on the home's interior.

Mike's brother Ron and his wife, Cindy, visited for the first time in decades. Mike and Ron had been estranged for years, and I was happy for Mike to reconnect with his brother, but sadly, I'm not sure he knew who he was.

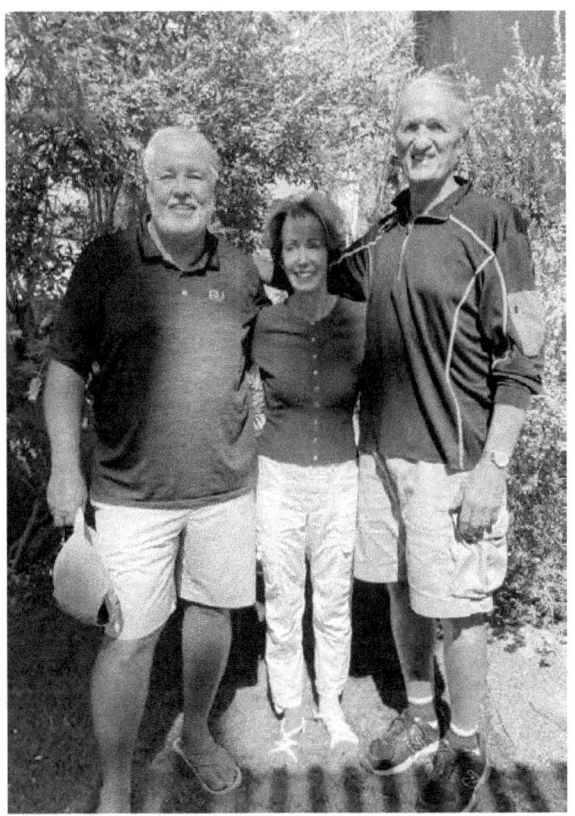

With brother Ron who visited us in Henderson

Scene 25

2022: Adventure World on the Seine

It was August, and the last European, or most likely last trip of any sort, was upon us. I was excited but felt like a tightrope walker about to perform without a net. *How would Mike react? Would he know we were going to Europe again? Would we have a repeat of previous trips where he was distraught because he was unfamiliar with the change in the environment?*

Since Mike and I would travel alone this time without the benefit of close relatives providing assistance, moral support, and companionship, I tried to reduce the stress on myself as much as possible. We still had Global Entry, which included TSAPre to speed us through the security and customs lines. I packed using only carry-on luggage—a first for me—and again used American Airlines' points to upgrade our flights to first class so he would be comfortable on the long flight.

I talked to him about the upcoming trip each day, and although he had repeatedly asked who would take care of Bijou, I was pretty sure he would be able to enjoy the vacation. I had trepidations, of course, but it was too late to back out. So, like a camper lost in the woods, I pressed forward, heading deeper and deeper into the dark forest.

The day of the flight had arrived, and Tom and Cathe dropped us off at the airport. Once inside the terminal with Mike and the luggage, I suddenly realized I was alone in this endeavor. I hadn't expected or fully appreciated the physical, emotional, and mental toll traveling with Mike in his current state would take on me—constantly helping him in unfamiliar places, starting at check-in at the airport.

It was like traveling with twin two-year-olds, a dog, and two cats. Getting boarding passes with passports, COVID-19 vaccination cards, ID at the kiosks, and going through customs while keeping my eye on him and the carry-ons was all a bit of a struggle—tip of the hat to single parents traveling with toddlers. Fortunately, unlike a toddler, Mike was a two-million miler with American Airlines, and we had upgraded to first class, so we got some special attention, assistance, and the use of the Executive Club.

While progressing through the terminal, I realized I couldn't leave Mike alone. We were one unit, stuck together for the duration. I felt like Blanche Dubois in *A Streetcar Named Desire*, relying on the kindness of strangers. "Excuse me, sir, my husband has dementia. Would you please walk with him into the men's room and direct him to a stall?"

Turning to Mike, I'd say, "Okay, follow that man. I'll wait right here." When I needed to use the restroom, I'd find a bench within eyesight of the entryway and tell him to sit right there until I returned. If a kind-looking person was nearby, I might ask her to "keep an eye" on him in case he got anxious. However, it became more manageable once we'd reached the American Airlines' Executive Club. We could sit, relax, dine, enjoy a glass of champagne, and use the facilities there while waiting for the flight.

The first-class seats from Chicago to Paris on British Airways—partner with AA—would have thrilled most people with a fully functioning brain. They differed from the old-style lounge chairs that reclined and were arranged side by side. Instead, we had our own cocoon-like console that lay completely flat for sleeping. These cone-shaped booths have a personal TV that hangs just above one's midsection when fully reclined.

I was ecstatic, anticipating reclining in the comfort of my cocoon with my audio-visual system, enjoying a glass of wine, and then stretching out and sleeping for six hours. What I hadn't realized, however, was that to someone with dementia, these boxes were frightening. Mike didn't know where we were, where we were going, or why we were lying in coffins. And he couldn't see me tucked away right next to us when we were lying flat.

Before the cabin lights went out, he would frequently call my name, and I would wave and say, "Here I am." However, he'd become distraught once it was dark. If he dozed off after holding my disembodied hand, he would not recognize where he was when he awoke, and he was terrified, shouting for me. This, of course, did not endear us to our fellow passengers.

Mike woke frequently. Each time he yelled, I sat up abruptly, exited my bed, and walked down to the crossover to the opposite aisle to help guide him to the large, handicapped bathroom. Fortunately, it was roomy enough for two, and I could direct him to the toilet paper, flusher, and sink to wash his hands. This went on multiple times during the night. I don't think he needed to use the restroom; he just needed the reassurance that I hadn't forsaken him. Neither of us got much sleep during the nearly nine-hour flight. *Well,* I thought, *that was a colossal waste of money—or points.* We would have gotten more rest scrunched up like pretzels back in coach.

Arriving at Charles de Gaulle Airport, I guided him through the immigration process and security and then to the arrival area, where a Viking employee greeted us. I felt like someone lost in the desert alone who finally saw another human being. I wasn't going to let him out of my sight.

Trying to keep up with the fast-moving guide carrying our bags, I trailed behind him with Mike following me. He had difficulty keeping me in sight, although I stayed just ten feet ahead and wore a bright-yellow shirt. "Sherry, Sherry," he'd call out every few yards like a blind man searching for his seeing-eye dog. I slowed down and held his hand.

When I passed a handicapped bathroom we could use together, I signaled the guide, and we went in. Getting out was more difficult. When we tried to leave, the lock had spun completely and uselessly in my hand, trapping us inside the small bathroom. We both experienced a few seconds of panic, but I tried deep breaths. Fortunately, our Viking guide knew we'd gone in, heard us banging on the door, and quickly extricated us. He was not about to lose two of his flock before herding us safely to the ship. By the time we had boarded, I was exhausted and almost ready to go home.

As I should have predicted, Mike was confused about where we were during the first few nights on board the vessel. He kept asking me to go home and see Bijou. I explained repeatedly that we were now in Europe, thousands of miles away, on a ship on a river.

He once again had trouble with the unfamiliar surroundings of the stateroom and bathroom. On the third day, however, it finally seemed to seep into his brain that we were on a boat far from home, and Bijou was staying with my sister. He relaxed, or at least quit asking about her.

Our fellow Viking passengers were delightful and kind. Realizing that Mike had dementia—because besides being observable, I readily shared this information—many made it a point to greet Mike daily and ask how we were doing. The attention pleased him, and he seemed to enjoy the rest of the cruise.

The highlight was a bicycle tour through Giverny to Monet's house and gardens. We met the tour guides at the dock, where they had thirty or forty bikes lined up for us to choose from. The Viking staff was skeptical about Mike's ability to ride the distance and tried to dissuade us from going, but I reassured them. "He'll be fine," I said, and he was. It was one of his best days.

We had selected a bike for him and ensured he could ride it as he circled the area, smiling broadly and waving. Muscle memory took over. We biked down paths and through a canopy of trees, admiring the charming city of Giverny, to arrive at Claude Monet's house. We walked through the beautiful mansion with his paintings displayed and through the lush gardens with lily ponds and bridges encircling the home. Despite the initial concerns of the Viking staff, Mike enjoyed the day as much as any he had experienced in the past few years. The day was mystical, or at least magical.

When we docked for the Normandy beaches tour, I had decided we didn't need to see them again. I would have liked to have seen the

English Cemetery we had signed up for since we had visited the American Cemetery twice before, but unfortunately, the beaches, I learned, were a two-hour coach ride from the ship. I didn't think Mike would enjoy the ride or understand where we were headed, so I opted for us to stay and stroll the surrounding, tree-lined paths along the river. It was both relaxing and beautiful.

Overall, it was a pleasant trip, but certainly not as much fun for me as it would have been only five years earlier when Mike could have fully conversed and shared the experience with me, chatting over dinner about the day's events. Our roles had certainly changed as I had transitioned from loving partner to loving caregiver.

The flights from Europe back to the US with the same cocoon beds were just as stressful for us as those from the US to Europe. Mike failed to remember them, and I felt a sense of déjà vu. We made it to Dallas, only to discover that bad weather had created hours of delays for the trip's second leg, which only added to my angst. Then, after waiting in the Executive Lounge for four hours, the flight was finally called, and we made our way to the gate.

Clutching our British Airways' first-class boarding passes, we stood with the first group and approached the computer. When our boarding passes were not recognized, the gate attendant looked at them and snatched them from my tired fingers. "Oh, they reassigned your seats," she said, laughing, and handed me two new ones.

"Thank you," I replied, not looking at them. After the transatlantic flight and long delays, I was exhausted, so I took the new boarding passes and we entered the plane. As I searched for the assigned seats at the front of the aircraft, I discovered they had unceremoniously dumped us in coach. The first-class seats on this domestic leg of the trip were the ample, old-style, extra legroom, side-by-side kind that Mike would have been much more comfortable sitting in.

I voiced my protest. They apologized. They did not provide any explanation, however, despite reserving those seats months ago. The flight attendants blamed the gate attendants. And if the cabin doors hadn't been locked, the gate attendants would likely have blamed the flight attendants. I guessed that due to all the delays and flight cancellations, they had overbooked first-class tickets, and the AA passengers outranked the BA passengers, so we got tossed out like the thirteenth and fourteenth eggs in a carton. So much for airline partnerships.

Exhausted after a long trip, I decided not to press it further, not wanting to get hauled off the plane in handcuffs. We were only a few hours from home, so I just closed my eyes and wished for ruby red slippers so, like Dorothy, I could click my heels together. *There's no place like home*, I thought.

After we returned to Henderson and looked through the photo book of the week that I had created online, Mike frequently said, "That was a fun trip." I smiled and nodded, thinking fun was probably not the adjective I would use. It would probably be our last trip anywhere. He enjoyed looking at the book for months and remembering some of it. He even noticed ads on TV for Viking cruises and pointed and smiled.

I was glad we went. I was happier we were home.

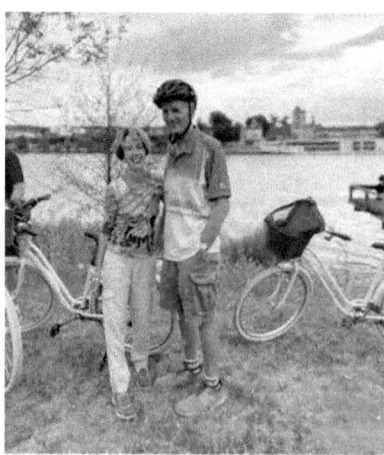

Biking to Monet's Garden. Best day

Scene 26
2023: Five Years After Diagnosis

Besides his growing inability to understand language, Mike now struggled with problem-solving and understanding concepts. His mental decline had been gradual, and, like a child growing up, it was impossible to see changes daily.

I measured it by looking back through the years. I charted Mike's regress as if we were tracking a child's progress—only in reverse. What skill could he manage last year that is beyond his reach now? Until five years ago, he could still drive a car alone. He could drive with me in the car until three years ago. And now, he's completely unable to drive at all. This had nothing to do with language and was only partly due to memory loss. Two years ago, he could still do expert sudoku, but gradually, the damnable Ratt ate that part of his brain, too, and today, the puzzle puzzles him. He stared at the squares in the newspaper, apparently not understanding what it was, much less how to solve it.

His dementia may have started with problems with memory and understanding words, but Ratt had burrowed in beyond that. Keeping Mike occupied is challenging when we're not bowling or walking Bijou. TV didn't hold his attention for long, so I tried games.

I bought a big, plastic tic-tac-toe board with big Xs and Os, but I was stunned when I discovered he could not grasp the concept of putting three similar objects in a row. He could not assemble a simple jigsaw puzzle designed for toddlers despite my help and the fact that it had less than ten pieces. He stared at the odd cutouts, unable to figure out what he was supposed to do with them. I tried large coloring books, but he was not interested, and when I showed him how to color in a square and handed him the crayon, he made check marks on the page. This was so far beyond language or simple memory problems.

Puzzle-solving is a very complex, cognitive process, I learned. It involves several brain regions that must work together to process and integrate information as the electrical impulses that the neurons send travel across the intricate roadway system.

The *prefrontal cortex,* at the front of the brain near the forehead—Mr. Big—is responsible for executive function, decision-making, and problem-solving. Near the brain's center, the *parietal lobe* plays a critical role in processing spatial information, including mental imagery, attention, and spatial reasoning. The *temporal lobe,* located on both sides of the brain, is responsible for processing auditory information, including language and memory. The *medial temporal lobe*, inside the temporal lobe near the brain's forward base, specifically the *hippocampus*, is involved in episodic memory, spatial navigation, and the formation of new memories. This lobe connects to the *occipital and parietal lobes.*[1] However, the primary function of the medial temporal lobe is to store and categorize declarative memory, including factual knowledge and personal memory. It also functions as a critical rest stop before memories can be moved to our long-term memory.[2] Every single one of these brain regions must work together under Mr. Big's direction to exchange information so that we can solve puzzles.

While Mr. Big tries to manage the lobes under his control, Ratt, in Mike's brain, is busy disrupting the highway of neurons that connects Mr. Big to his subordinates. I wondered if that meant that the damage had

---

1. gameslearningsociety.org/.

2. Scienceabc.com.

progressed to Mike's frontal lobe or that the damaged lobes could not connect with Mr. Big in the frontal lobe. Either way, their communication was disrupted, resulting in Mike's inability to solve puzzles or think critically. Despite the many discoveries about the brain, scientists are still working to unravel the great mysteries of the human body's most complex organ.

Music, also once a big part of Mike's life, didn't interest him any longer, except for watching some music videos or performances on *America's Got Talent* (AGT). It's the visual, not the sound, he is interested in. In fact, he wanted the sound to be turned down low. Loud noises now bothered him, and if the volume was too noisy, he covered his ears and made a frightened face as if a firecracker had just exploded on the coffee table.

Music enjoyment is housed in the temporal lobe, where the perception of sound is located. Perhaps another PET scan would show the progression of the damage. I made a mental note to ask Simrit on the next visit to Lou Ruvo.

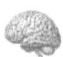

Since Mike preferred being at home when we weren't bowling or walking the dog, I started thinking about a caregiver–companion who could stay with Mike for a few hours each time while I ran errands or had lunch with a friend. The end of July was set as the publication date for my second book, *Mac: The Wind Beneath My Wings*, which I expected would require time away from home for promotional activities and book signings.

It was time to call Unum, our long-term care provider. Mike did not need help with "Activities of Daily Living," which is generally a prerequisite to activating the policy. He just couldn't be left alone for over an hour because he was incapable of seeking help in an emergency. He also would feel panicky if left alone for too long. Unum scheduled a Zoom meeting with a third-party agency, and the woman asked Mike questions he could neither understand nor respond to. This clearly showed them that he—or rather I—qualified for assistance, and they activated the policy.

A bubbly woman named Miranda was sent by the Home Instead agency I'd called. She was quite a character. Although born in the Philippines, she hailed from Barcelona, Spain, and brought to mind Carmen Miranda, the 1940s rumba dancer. She had a charming accent and talked incessantly. Miranda was in her early seventies and dressed as if she was stopping by the house on her way to a cocktail party. She wore heavy makeup and thick, false eyelashes. I expected to hear the clack-clack of castanets each time she walked through the front door.

The agency's minimum four-hour period was too long for Mike, who did not enjoy being left with Miranda. When I returned after the first time, he gave me an angry look and said, "I had nothing to do." Of course, he would have had nothing to do if I had been there, but being left alone with a stranger for four hours was entirely different. I also think my absence made him acutely aware of his limitations and lack of freedom.

Still, I wanted to go out twice a week for a couple of hours while he was safe at home with a caregiver, so I whittled the time down to three hours twice a week with the agency, which they said was their absolute minimum. Instead of working out at home, I joined the Las Vegas Athletic Club and enjoyed using their well-equipped gym, swimming in the indoor pool, and having lunch between workouts. I could also run errands and occasionally get my nails and hair done.

Miranda laughed when she told me that the last hour before I returned, Mike said, "Where's Sherry? She's been gone six years."

"Yes," I said, smiling. "He confuses the words."

Each time I'd left, Mike was miserable. When I returned, he glared at me angrily and went to pout in his bedroom. I had hoped he would, in time, get used to Miranda and realize I would return in a couple of hours, but he never did.

About six months after she had first started coming, I walked up to Mike after breakfast as he sat in his chair, watching a football game replayed, and said slowly, as I did each time, "I am going to the gym this morning." I paused. "Then I am going to the grocery store. I will be back at 2:00." I held up two fingers. "Miranda will be here to make your lunch." I repeated this two more times until I felt he understood I was going to go out.

His eyes filled with tears. "You do this all the time," he stammered. "You go and have fun. I am here. What do *I* do?"

Then the doorbell rang, and Bijou barked.

"Already?" he said. Again, his eyes filled with tears. I let Miranda in and went back to Mike. I began the explanation I went through each Tuesday and Thursday: "You don't want to go on errands with me. I took you to the gym and showed you. You said that you don't want to go."

He pursed his lips in an expression that said, "You don't understand."

Oh, but I do, I thought. *I just wish that I could change your situation.*

"I only go for a couple of hours," I said, defending myself. "I will be back at 2:00, and then we can go to the park or bowl if you want." I know he can't understand most of my words. He only knows that I am leaving. I know he feels abandoned, that I feel guilty, and I ache for him. His frustration is evident. Whenever I leave, it is a bitter reminder that he has lost his independence. He could not go out even if there was somewhere that he wanted to go. He has been left behind by me, by fate, by life.

"Just go," he said, waving me away with his hand.

I kissed him on the forehead. "I love you. I will be back in a couple of hours." Then I grabbed my gym bag and the picture frame I was taking to be repaired and walked to the car.

I sat behind the wheel for a few minutes and rethought this situation. I hated going through this twice a week. I felt drained. I tossed ideas around in my head like a game of catch as I reasoned and bickered with myself. Should I call the agency and tell them I want to cancel the service? I could take him wherever I went on errands, but then I remembered my workouts.

I could go back to working out at home. I have most of the weights and could buy more. What about aerobics? When I joined the athletic club, I gave away the broken indoor bike that took up space in the bedroom. I have a pool at home, but it's really only usable in the summer.

Back and forth, pro and con, I argued with myself, throwing ideas out and then back in again. Finally, I concluded it was only a few hours twice a week. He wants to be with me, but he wants me to be at home. I must go out occasionally to the gym, get my nails done, and run errands. I spend every other waking hour with him. It's okay for me to leave for a few hours, I told myself. I just wish I didn't feel so guilty about it.

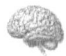

Five years had passed since Mike was diagnosed with dementia. His memory had, of course, faded in all areas. He understood fewer and fewer words and could not articulate many at all now. There was so much that he no longer understood. And, of course, I could not explain things to him because he couldn't understand what I was saying. He could only grasp the simplest of words. Yet, he talks to me when he needs something or wants to bring something to my attention.

Linguistically, Mike can't say the sound that the letter L makes and hasn't been able to for at least a year. Bijou is his little grrrrr. He said why for the word while, as in "We haven't done that in a why." It's the L sound he can't pronounce. But also, he said "right nigh" for right now. He doesn't know the names of many everyday objects. He continually hums softly or chants curious clauses. Brr burr quac quac quac, particularly when he is anxious. Conversation is impossible, but he still says many phrases, such as, "Where's the dog? Look at clouds. Ears dead," and even, "I'm looking forward to bowling." Anything more complicated is garbled.

He still wants to take Bijou for a walk alone, but today, he got lost. The neighbors brought him home, so I bought a GPS for Bijou's collar. It wouldn't help Mike navigate his world, but at least I could track their progress on my iPhone when they were out. And he could continue to walk with her to one of the two parks in the neighborhood.

At this point, Mike rarely understood me when I asked him questions, and sometimes, he looked in the wrong direction when I called him. He couldn't remember to take his medications out of the pillbox, so I handed them to him and waited while he swallowed them. He was unable to make his lunch anymore, forgetting where everything was stored and probably how to make a sandwich.

But clearly, Mike thought about lots of things and made observations. Every other Wednesday, the house cleaners come while we are bowling and are occasionally there when we return. He sat and watched them while I worked on the computer. Afterward, at dinner that evening, he was quiet for a long time. Then he looked up. "Those grrrsss. The peeep. They do hard." His head tilts in admiration.

"Yes," I said, understanding. "The housekeepers work very hard. They do a great job."

"How long work?"

"They're here four hours. They work very hard." He mulled that over, nodding.

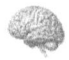

BD (before dementia), Mike was meticulous about grooming and showered daily. This year, he didn't grasp the point unless we were going to go bowling or to the doctor's office, and even then, he didn't see the need. I understood. He didn't do much to work up a sweat. The only time that he automatically took a shower was after sex, so sometimes I initiated sex just to get him into the shower. It was a win–win situation.

Other than that, I insisted he shower at least every other day. "You shower?" he asked me accusingly, as if he were being asked to do something strange and out of the ordinary.

"Yes, I just took my shower." He looked at me skeptically. I learned to take my shower first, walk out in a towel, and show him my wet hair. "See? I have taken my shower. Now it's your turn." This way, he didn't feel that he was being singled out for water torture punishment.

I then treated it like a game. I pointed at his armpits, pinched my nose, and said, "Stinky." He laughed, and I danced toward the bathroom, pulling him gently. I coaxed his T-shirt off, told him to sit on the bed, and removed his shoes.

Then he lowered his pants and stepped out of them after reminding me to close the shades to prevent Peeping Toms. He became very concerned about voyeurs who might be lurking outside our house. These determined, depraved individuals would first have to target our home, which sits at the end of a cul-de-sac with no houses directly across the street. Then they would need to enter our fenced front yard, move stealthily around the fronds of a large palm tree, and peer under the half-open sunshade to look into his bedroom. *Unlikely,* I thought, but I lowered the blinds to appease him. Then I led him into the bathroom. This process took a little more time but created less stress for both of us.

Once undressed, I laid his clean underwear and socks on the bathroom vanity, reminding him to take out his hearing aids, and I watched while he removed them. He took off his watch and ring, which he wore daily, and stepped into the shower. I pointed at the shampoo/body wash, and he nodded, making a face, sometimes annoyed that I was reminding him. He showered, toweled off, and donned his clean underwear and socks. I, of course, peeked in occasionally and came in when he was ready to head into the bedroom to finish dressing.

Physically, Mike is still incredibly fit. His pacemaker completely regulates his erratic tachycardia. He wears a hearing aid, but aside from that, he is physically healthy. When he undresses, I still can't help but admire his lean, athletic body. He has never been overweight but has lost muscle in his once-powerful legs and arms. He stands tall, with no bow in his shoulders, with the body of a much younger man.

In some ways, things are easier for me now. I don't have to ask what Mike wants for dinner or if he wants to go out. He eats whatever I serve him and goes wherever I take him. We don't battle over which shows to watch on TV. Whatever I choose, he stares at for a few minutes before he loses focus.

In other ways, however, many things are more challenging. He wants to feel useful and still participate in life and in our partnership, which has become an additional activity for me. A few months ago, he would look for the two canisters in the house where I keep recyclables and automatically take them to the big, blue recycle bin on the side of the house. When he forgot where it was, I moved the can into the garage to make it easier for him to access, but soon, he forgot where it was in the garage. Then I handed the containers to him, and he usually asked, "Where do you want these?"

"In the blue can in the garage," I replied. He looked puzzled. Either he could not understand the word garage, or he had forgotten where the garage was. "I'll show you." Then we went together, I pointed out the can, and he emptied the smaller container into the larger one. This meant, of course, that I had to stop what I was doing to help him do the task that I could just as easily have done myself and in less time. It would have been less stressful, but he needed things to do to feel useful.

My arms were full of things I wanted to put in the box for Goodwill. "Can you open the garage door, honey?" I asked as I stood in front of it. Of course, this damage to his brain prevents him from understanding my words, but he frequently can't glean the meaning even with active pantomime.

"What?" he replied, staring blankly at me.

"Can you open the doooor," I said slowly, making a circle with my one free hand and pointing at the door.

"I don't know what you're talking about," he said, looking quizzical, and then walked away.

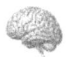

One Saturday in May, I decided to see if he could still enjoy golf, which he had always excelled at. We drove to a local course a few miles from the house. It was a beautiful day, and we walked to the driving range. I took out his driver, and we stood and watched other golfers hit some balls. I asked if he wanted to try it, but he demurred. "No," he said simply and smiled. He seemed to know what he was capable of doing and what he was not.

We walked to the putting green, and I handed him his putter. He and I used to have putting contests occasionally at cocktail time on the putting green we had installed in the backyard of our Las Flores house after the grandsons outgrew the jungle gym and sandpit.

"Putt the ball in that hole like this," I said as I demonstrated with a crowd-pleasing, six-foot shot into the hole. He tried a few times but didn't seem to understand the concept of directing the small, white sphere into the hole. He'd punch at the ball, putting it nowhere near the cup.

After fifteen or twenty minutes of halfhearted, unsuccessful attempts, we gave up and enjoyed a glass of wine on the patio, watching the golfers. He chatted amiably with the servers. A casual observer might not be able to tell that he had dementia at this point. Deep thought and discussions were beyond him, but he could communicate adequately with small talk, for the most part.

As I thought about this day later, I realized we hadn't golfed in several years. This was something he had enjoyed his entire adult life. As he tapered off, he had complained that his shoulder hurt too much to swing a club. *Why bowling and not golf?* I wondered. Then I reasoned that golf differs from bowling in many ways.

With golf, the brain needs to gather data, make decisions, and figure out what shot should be played and which club should be used to accomplish the task. Though a good bowler must carefully consider where to place the ball to hit the correct spot, participating in bowling requires simply taking a few steps and throwing the ball at the pins. This was something Mike could still do. As long as he hit some, it was satisfying. Occasionally, he could exult over a spare or a strike. The margin for error in golf was much smaller and frustrating, even for those who had healthy brains.

Oddly, this summer, unlike all previous summers, he had no interest in going near the pool to swim, float on the rubber raft, or even lie on the lounge chair to warm himself for a few minutes as he used to do. I wondered if he was afraid that he couldn't remember how to swim or if it was due to increased damage in the parietal lobe that controls spatial relations. Navigating in the water could be frightening. For whatever reason, he preferred to stay in the safety of the house.

At dinner, Mike spoke very little, concentrating on his food with the careful deliberation of someone focused on a complex math equation. After dinner, he put his plates on the kitchen counter and tried to put things away, asking where the salt and pepper were kept. While he was "helping," I watched him like an eagle searching for prey because everything cold went into the freezer.

While preparing his ice cream dish, I found ketchup in the freezer. Our old refrigerator was a double door, with the freezer on the bottom and the fridge on the top. Our new refrigerator is side by side. The refrigerator is on the right, and the freezer is on the left. He could not understand or remember that the left side was now a freezer. To my horror and annoyance, I discovered several Diet Coke cans had exploded in the freezer as he tried to save a half-finished can. This is indeed a mess to clean up, but I need not have worried. Six months later, he could no longer remember to put anything away on either side of the refrigerator.

My second book, *Mac: The Wind Beneath My Wings*, was published on the 27th of July. It was an exhilarating time for me, but unfortunately, Mike couldn't share my accomplishments. He seemed to understand that I'd written another book as he looked at a picture or two. "I'll read," he said, smiling. But of course, he could no longer read.

At the urging and kind invitation of Cathe and Tom, I hosted a big book signing party at their larger house, with about fifty friends and relatives invited. It had everything: good food, fine wines and cold beers, and a large display of Mac's memorabilia and photos on the pool table. The only thing missing were books to sell and sign. Unfortunately, the first printing had ten misprinted pages where some of the footnotes appeared in the text of the book. So, while I could display them for the guests to ooh and aah over, there were no books for them to purchase, or for me to sign. I felt like Alice at the Mad Hatter's unbirthday party.

Much of Mike's distant past is no longer accessible to him, nor is the immediate past, but he has some memories in between. Yesterday, on the way to the dog park, we passed Chavelos Mexican Restaurant. "There's our place," he pointed out happily, although it had been several weeks since our last visit. He remembered it. He will also see an ad for Viking River Cruises on the television and say, "We did that." But much of the past is gone—short and long-term memories.

Just as the past is fading, there are no long-term future thoughts, either, but I suppose that's good. He does not dwell on what the future might bring or when. He lives in the now and enjoys what he can. He sometimes reflects on the day, "This was a busy day" or "This was a good day," and smiles. "Bowl tomorrow?" but that was as far into the future as he could envision. Mike has always been the embodiment of someone who lives in the moment. But now, it seemed, he was imprisoned by the present.

Even though he had nothing to do but sit in his chair, Mike was most comfortable at home and did not enjoy going places unless it was for bowling. This included riding in the car to go on errands. Taking him with me when I needed to make three or four quick stops added time and increased my stress and his. Sometimes, he was still fine staying home alone with the dog, and I could leave him for up to an hour. At the beginning of the year, he could still use his senior flip phone to call me if needed, and he was not a wandering risk, nor did he try to cook anything, so I didn't worry about his safety. He sat in his La-Z-Boy chair and stared at the TV screen.

Sometime midyear, I realized he could no longer use his phone, so I discontinued his phone service and recycled his flip phone. He stared at it as though he didn't even recognize what it was—and maybe he didn't. Once the possibility of communicating with me ended when I was out, he no longer wanted to stay by himself for any length of time.

I had joined a group of local authors who held book signings at various coffee shops and senior independent living establishments, and I signed up for one about every two weeks. However, by the end of the year, I had to give them up. It was fun getting out, talking with folks, and selling a few books, but in the end, the three or four hours required were not worth the time I had spent. Mike did not cope well with being left with a caregiver while I was gone for half a day, nor did he take to sitting with me in a coffee shop for the duration. The most productive and enjoyable event I'd participated in was a PowerPoint presentation I gave to an audience of two hundred veterans. Those events were rare, and soon, I just quit trying to set them up, instead concentrating on spending time with Mike and writing this book.

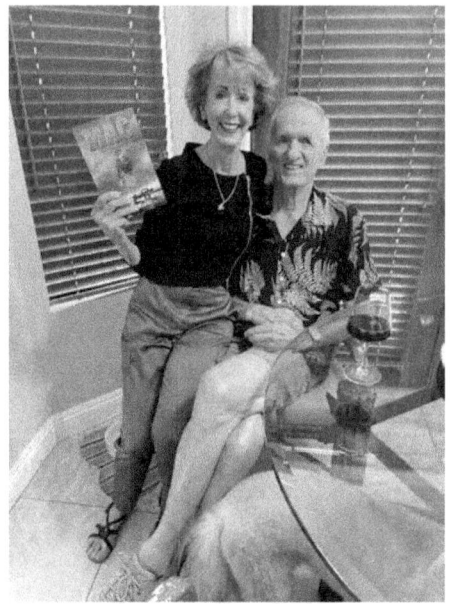

Celebrating MAC at the unsigning party

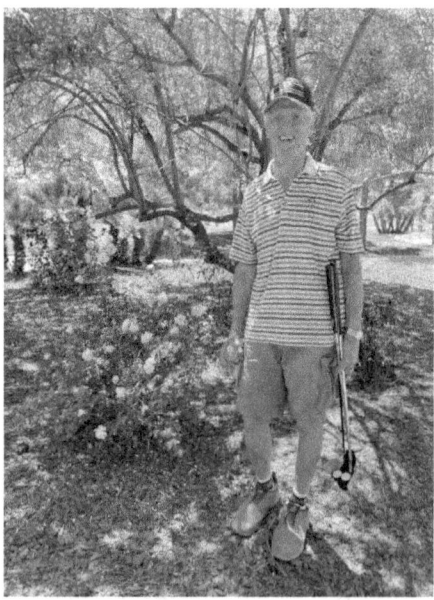

Trying to remember playing golf

Scene 27
Mike and Bijou

After each walk, Bijou zoomed around the dining room table with a toy tossed in between and barked for her treats, which I handed to Mike to dispense. He mimed that he was not hungry—joking—then happily provided them to her while sitting in his armchair, laughing at her antics. I handed him the treats so he could interact with her since he no longer knew where they were stored.

Even though Bijou knows I am now "the leader of the pack," she is still devoted to him. She came to me for food, water, and treats if Mike didn't respond to her pleas, but she kissed him awake in the morning and sat on the arm of his chair frequently when he stared at the television. He and Bijou are very connected.

Mike still found great comfort in *his* dog, Bijou, and constantly worried about her. "Where's my dog?" he'd asked me multiple times daily.

"She's here somewhere." I sighed. "She's sleeping." Together, we'd make an expedition to find out which of her many retreats she was currently located in. Satisfied that she was alive and well, he relaxed until the next time he remembered to ask.

Mike had forgotten Bijou's name. It's doggy or my dog. He sometimes called Bijou "doctor." Even in his stage of dementia, I am sure he knows she did not go to medical school or get an advanced degree. "Where's the doctor?" he asked repeatedly, looking under beds.

Miranda called me a little distraught one day as I left the grocery store. "Sherry, Mike is rubbing his chest where the pacemaker is and asking for the doctor. I'm worried."

"I'll be right there," I said. Then I realized he was asking about the dog. Rubbing his chest was unrelated to the question about the doctor.

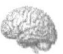

Mike continued to moan softly when he was anxious, usually when we went to a doctor's appointment or bowling and left Bijou at home. "Where's the dog? Alone?" he asked with a frightened look on his face.

"No, house cleaners are there," I said, as they are every other Wednesday while we bowl, and I reminded him on those occasions. This alleviated his anxiety. He sighed.

"They like him?"

"Yes," I assured him. "They love her."

"They're there with him? Oh, that's so nice," he said, relieved, as if the house cleaners had come solely to stay with Bijou and keep her company while we were bowling.

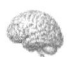

Bijou still jumped on his bed each morning, awakening him with gentle doggie kisses. I sat in the living room, reading the morning paper and drinking coffee, smiling as I listened to him happily talking to her in the bedroom. They speak the same language, and they seem to understand each other. Then he'd get up, and they'd go for a walk.

I felt comfortable when they were out as I followed their progress around the neighborhood on my iPhone through the GPS. Mike still insisted on taking her for morning walks, but the distance became shorter as he feared going too far afield. Of course, he did not know that I could monitor their whereabouts.

Bijou turned twelve this year. The dog was a familiar friend, and Mike clung to her. Unfortunately, she had picked up anxious behaviors, trying to cope with Mike's changing demeanor.

I learned to wait until she whined to be fed, or she would ignore it until it was crusty and had to be discarded. When she signaled she was ready to begin the eating ritual, I put her food down and she approached it cautiously—stalking the bowl of dog food like wild prey. Then she spent several minutes nudging imaginary dirt over the bowl in an attempt to cover it from potential pack rivals, I assume, that might drag it off into the bush.

She pulled the little mat under the dish over her food and sometimes shoved the bowl under the table, trying to hide it. She wanted me to put the food down, but she wasn't necessarily ready to eat it. Moments later, she realized she was hungry and came into my office to bark at me.

"I fed you, you silly girl," I told her. "You covered it up." Then together, we went to the bowl, which I uncovered, and sprinkled the food with cheese. She slowly meandered over and ate, giving me the side-eye, as if she was doing me a big favor as she nibbled the food delicately. Pleased with herself afterward, she ran circles in the dining room or raced up and down the hallway, expecting a treat for her incredible, food-disappearing magic act. And, of course, I rewarded her performance.

Bijou also seemed to understand that Mike couldn't fend for himself any longer, so she took it upon herself to ensure I fed him in a timely manner. Even though she had eaten by 5:00, she came to find me and barked. This was her way of telling me it was time for me to go to the kitchen and make dinner for Mike. She is not abandoning him, even if she thinks that I have.

On Sunday, we made our afternoon trek to the park. Because Mike rarely walked Bijou in the morning now, each afternoon this past summer, when the temperatures were over one hundred degrees, I loaded the dog and

Michael into the car and drove two and a half miles to Fox Ridge Park. It's a bit larger than a football field and lined with trees. The gigantic pines provided a lovely, shaded stroll, and the occasional breeze made even the 90-to-115-degree weather tolerable.

As we pulled up to the park this time, Mike told me his hearing aid battery was dead. I carry extra batteries, so whenever this happens, I motion for him to take the device out and hand it to me. It usually takes a few minutes and some dramatic pantomimes on my part before he understands what I am asking. When I have it, I tap it on my ear to see if it is pinging or if the battery is indeed dead. As we stepped onto the park grass, he told me again, "Dead."

"Hand it to me," I pantomimed, holding out my hand. Finally, he took it out of his ear, and I plucked it from his palm and put it to my ear. The battery pinged loudly. "Good," I pronounced. "Put it back in."

I placed it in his hand, and at that moment, I thought, *We should not be standing on the grass. We should move to the sidewalk.* Too late. He opened his hand, slowly letting the hearing aid slide down and drop in the grass. I gasped in horror. This would not be the first one that he had lost. The last one was found only because he'd crushed it to smithereens while we hunted for it. They cost over three thousand dollars.

"Don't move," I commanded, and of course, he immediately stepped back, still holding Bijou's leash. Now, I rushed to pinpoint the spot where he had been standing. If all things were right in the universe, it should be lying on the top of the grass right below where his feet had been. I got down on my hands and knees and searched. Nothing. "Back away," I directed. He was totally oblivious. Bijou began to whine. We had arrived at the park, but we weren't walking anywhere, she must have thought. The temperature was 110 degrees.

"What are you doing?" Mike yelled angrily.

"Your hearing aid. You dropped your hearing aid. I am looking for it," I screamed back at him. He watched me curiously for a few minutes as I rooted about in the grass, and then he grew hot and tired of standing there holding the dog's leash. "Go. Come on, come on," he yelled repeatedly, not understanding what I had been doing on my hands and knees, scraping the grass for the past twenty minutes.

"I'm looking for your damn hearing aid," I shouted back. But of course, he couldn't understand me. He continued to yell, telling me to come, as if I was somehow having fun playing in the grass, and he was ready to go. I wanted to leap up and pummel him.

After a few more minutes of his yelling, "Go," I marked the spot, and we went home. I called my sister, and she and I trekked back to the park while Tom sat with Mike at home.

After a half hour's search, I decided some squirrel must have a vast cache of hearing aids and sunglasses stored in a tree somewhere and told Cathe we should end the futile search in five minutes. After all, it was blast-furnace hot. At that moment, I had dug deep into a clump of grass and magically plucked it out. "Eureka! I found it," I yelled, then blew out a deep breath of air.

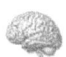

Months later, it was a crisp fall afternoon, so I decided we should walk to the park behind our house instead of driving to Fox Ridge Park. What a delightful outing it turned out to be. It was as if Mike was taking me on a tour of his old walking routes. He smiled, laughed, and constantly chatted as he pointed out familiar things. Some of his words were wrong, but I could easily decipher his meaning. "Beautiful day. No wind, that's the key," he'd repeated multiple times.

"Yes, it's a beautiful day," I responded.

"We went this way last year," he said, pointing in the opposite direction.

"Yes, you went to the small park this morning."

"Uh-huh." He smiled.

After a few steps, he pointed at a well-trimmed bush in a neighbor's yard. "Nice job." A few paces farther, he pointed at Bijou. "He know where to go. Leader." When Bijou squatted to relieve herself, Mike turned to me and reported, "Just a pee-pee. Two spots." A few steps farther, he pointed at the ground. "She poops here and there," indicating frequent duty stations. As we approached the playground, he pointed and beamed. "Kids," he tells me.

"Yes, it's fun seeing the kids play," I responded. He had developed a great joy in watching little children and delighted in observing the babies and toddlers.

We finally rounded the circular path, and he pointed at the back of our house, which abuts the park. "Our house," he said twice with obvious pride. We walked out of the park and back to our street. "Sky, warm. No wind. That's the key," he repeated. Nearing our house, he again said, "Home," and we were there. He was like a small child showing off his toys. I marveled at the pleasant experience and planned to make walking in the neighborhood a habit, weather permitting.

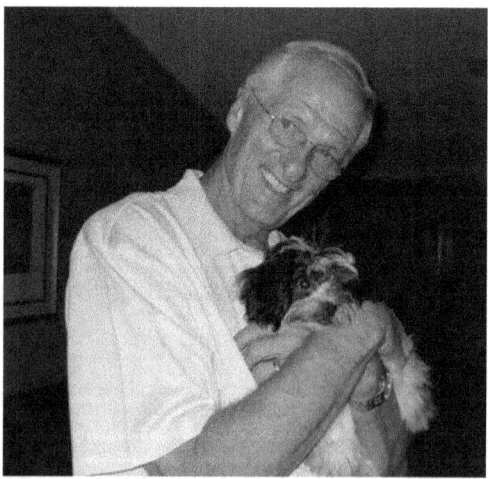

Mike and his buddy Bijou

Scene 28

2023: Autumn and Winter in AdventureWorld

I had repurchased the NFL package this year because Mike still enjoyed watching the Kansas City Chiefs play. When the preseason started, we looked forward to Sundays, Mondays, and Thursday evenings when he had something to watch. He was excited when the "Big Boys" played. I tried Saturday college games, but he had zero interest. "No," he moaned. "Not the Big Boys." I assumed the "Big Boys" meant the NFL instead of college teams. But sometimes, even when an NFL game was on, he complained. "They are not the Big Boys." This back-and-forth exchange frustrated me.

"Yes, they are the Big Boys. It's the NFL," I yell. "They don't get any bigger than that."

"No. Not the Big Boys," he said with finality and a smirk that suggested I didn't know what I was talking about. This argument went on repeatedly, to my great annoyance.

I tried to watch most of the KC games with him, and strangely enough, after forty years of not watching football, I became a semi-fan of the Chiefs. Knowing something about the personalities and love lives of Mahomes and Kelce helped keep my interest. The funny thing was that I found myself explaining rudimentary football plays to Mike. "The other team intercepted the ball, honey. Now they have the ball and will try to score. And now, they will kick for a field goal because they are running out of tries for a first down to keep the ball and score a touchdown. But they are in range to score three points."

"Uh-huh." He nodded, not understanding a single thing that I'd said. For my part, I was rather impressed with my vast football knowledge. The twenty-five-year-old Mike would have been so proud of me.

On Monday night, we watched the Cincinnati Bengals play the Jacksonville Jaguars. It was a great game. With eight minutes remaining in the fourth quarter, both teams were tied with a score of 28 to 28. Mike looked bored and uninterested. "Do you want to go to bed?" I asked.

"I'll watch the Big Boys tomorrow."

Me, slapping my head. "These *are* the Big Boys. This is Monday Night Football—the NFL. Tomorrow is Tuesday. Nobody plays football on Tuesday, Mike. ARRRGGGG!" I took a breath. "Okay, it's all tied up. Why don't you go to bed, and I'll record it?"

"Yes. Tomorrow, the Big Boys play."

"NOOOOO. THESE *ARE* THE BIG BOYS!" Then it dawned on me. After months of arguments trying to interest Mike in an NFL game—and with him stubbornly refusing to watch it because they are not the "Big Boys"—I realized that the "Big Boys" were not the NFL but the Kansas City Chiefs. That was the only game in town as far as he was concerned.

As understanding dawned, I took a deep breath. "Mike, Kansas City does not play tomorrow. There is no game on Tuesday."

He gave me a wry smile as if to say, "You'll see," then headed to his bedroom.

Mike is no longer interested in watching any other sport on TV. He, of course, played basketball, baseball, tennis, and golf most of his life and enjoyed watching them on TV. Now, only the Kansas City Chiefs and Patrick Mahomes, as he performs his magic, interested him.

As the season progressed, I realized he was not interested in other NFL teams and couldn't follow the entire game regardless of who it was. Sometimes, if I was writing in the other room, I would check on him and discover that he had wandered away from the TV. When I asked why, he told me that the game was over. After checking the screen, I said, "No, seven minutes are left in the third quarter." He could neither stay focused on the game nor read the score, and I wondered how much of the play he now understood.

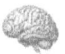

On November 8, our first great-grandchild was born. Corben and Lauryn blessed us with yet another boy in the family, Coa Carter Hobbs. The timing was not ideal for them because Lauryn was in a rigorous PhD program in psychology, and Corben was in his second year as a speech therapist, getting ready to start his master's program. But is the timing ever perfect for bringing children into the world? Money was tight, and the three of them moved in with her mother to help make ends meet, with all three sharing babysitting duties.

Life happens, as they say, when you are making plans, and some of life's most rewarding events occur when they are not planned. Corben and Lauryn have learned that going with the flow of the river of life is much easier than fighting the current, and they approached this momentous event with love, gratitude, and much joy.

As the birth neared, my first inclination was to drive to Southern California to see them. As I started making plans in my head, I realized it would be a nightmare of a trip. Mike would not know where we were going or understand why. Everything would be unfamiliar again at a hotel, so I had decided that our traveling days were over. In addition, the new parents and baby would probably enjoy some alone time.

They were blessed with multiple sets of parents, grandparents, and even great-grandparents who lived nearby. Coa even has a great-great-grandmother, Juanita, and great-great-grandfather, Lynn, who are in their late nineties. I decided that the new family could do without an early visit from the three of us. While we wouldn't see the grands and great-grand for the holidays, they would visit us shortly thereafter.

Of course, Mike could not feel the excitement or even understand what had happened to whom. His fascination with babies, in general, though, made him smile when he saw pictures of Coa or we FaceTimed, even if he didn't understand that he was the baby's great-grandfather.

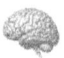

We went to sister Cathe and Tom's house on Thanksgiving as usual. I did not expect Mike to behave strangely, but with dementia, I had learned to expect the unexpected. We had always taken Bijou when we went to their house, and even though this required us to leave the sanctity of our home, we were only traveling one hundred yards to a place Mike was very familiar with.

Because I contributed a few dishes to the family gathering, I packed Bijou, Mike, and the food into my car and we drove down eight houses. I did not take Bijou's leash because she would happily jump out of the car and run into their home. We followed her, and at the door, Mike picked her up and held her. "Happy Thanksgiving!" I yelled as we walked into the foyer.

The whole family—my brother, Derreck, who was living with Cathe and Tom, their son, Devon, who lived across the street with his son, Chance, and his daughter, Abby, who was home from college—was already there. Tom's brother John, whose apartment is within walking distance, also joined the family.

As we stood in the entryway, Mike held Bijou tightly, not wanting to put her down. She usually had the run of the house and frolicked with their dog, Gobi, but not on this day. Mike stood there, cradling her protectively. When we sat down to eat, he wouldn't let go of the dog or eat Thanksgiving dinner, shaking his head and motioning that he wasn't hungry. When I handed him a piece of ham to taste, he took it off the fork and gave it to Bijou.

After the family had finished eating, he stood holding the dog, pointing at the door, and growled, "Go home." After a few minutes, we took some leftovers and drove the one hundred yards home. I heated the food and tried to get him to eat, but he wouldn't. Then he went to his bedroom, got into his bed, and pulled the covers over his face.

Concerned, I followed him and lay down beside him in the dark. It was only about 6:30. He brought my face close and kissed me repeatedly. *What did this mean?* I wondered. *Was this a silent protest? An apology for leaving the Thanksgiving dinner? Is he going to sleep and die in the night?* He finally stroked my cheek and smiled, indicating I could leave now. I kissed him, patted his head, and left the room. I sat in the living room sipping a glass of wine until I finally turned off the light and got into my bed to read. Even considering his dementia, I still couldn't explain his unusual behavior.

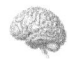

It's a Saturday, a cold December day. There is no league bowling at the Sunset or football on TV —at least not an NFL game. We walked with Bijou to the park, and afterward, as I was writing on my computer, I felt Mike standing in the doorway and turned toward him. He was pointing at his watch. "What do you need, babe?" I asked him. "It's not dinnertime yet; it's only four o'clock." I held up four fingers.

"I'm bore."

"I know you are," I said with a strained, sympathetic look on my face. "Do you want me to put a movie on?" I walked into the front room and said, "Free movie" into the Cox Cable channel changer microphone. Because he liked it and had seen it dozens of times over the years, I chose

A Christmas Story. I had hoped it might hold his interest and returned to the computer.

He was up in five minutes looking for lights to turn off or on, blinds to pull down, or trash to empty. "Okay, let's play catch." I pulled a white rubber ball from Bijou's cache, sat on the fireplace, and tossed it to him. He was delighted and made silly faces and gestures, obviously entertained for a few minutes. Then he put the ball down and made a face, conveying an expression that said, "Well, that's enough of that."

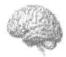

One night, late in December, we had the most extended dinner conversation that we'd had in a while. Of course it involved bowling. "Tomorrow?" he'd asked hopefully.

"Nope. No bowling for two weeks."

"That doesn't make sense," he said clearly and well-enunciated.

"It's Christmas and New Year's holiday," I told him. "But we can still go bowling, just not with the league."

"Hmmmm ... what tomorrow?"

"We can take a drive, the three of us."

He made a silly face. "Oh boy. That'll be fun! Yeah!" More silly faces. I laughed. Shades of the healthy brain "old days."

The following day, since the bowling leagues took a break during the holidays, I was desperate to find something for him to do, so we drove to Sunset Station to bowl—just the two of us. When we arrived, he looked around and asked, "Where people?"

"This is the holidays. No league bowling. Just you and I are going to bowl."

"What? No!" He scrunched his nose in displeasure.

"You don't want to bowl? I thought you missed bowling."

"No, no fun," he said. It suddenly hit me like a bowling ball to the headpin. It's not bowling, I realized. It's the competition he liked and the idea that he thought he would win some money.

Okay, I thought. *Since he doesn't want to bowl, this is a great time to try the game room.* I guided him into the area. "Let's play Skee-Ball," I said brightly with a big grin on my face. He looked at me blankly. I led him over to a machine and inserted the money. The balls rolled down the slide, and I picked one up. I rolled it up the slanted table, and it landed perfectly in the top circle.

"You try it," I urged, handing a ball to him. He looked at it, and after watching me make a throwing motion several times, he let go of the ball. It rolled slowly a few inches up the board and fell back into the trough. "Throw it harder," I said. He tried three or four more times but could not understand that he needed to throw it harder.

I gave up on Skee-Ball and moved to the air hockey game. I handed him a paddle, went to the other side of the table, and whacked the puck with my paddle. Mike stood as stiff as a marble statue and watched it go into the goal and disappear in front of him. I tried again, tapping it softly, trying to avoid the goal. When it reached his side of the table, I yelled, "Hit it!" He then hurled his paddle hard at the puck, sending both off the table.

I was glad that no small children were in the line of fire. I tried several more times to get him to hold on to the paddle and hit the ball, but it was fruitless. We left. I felt defeated. He was happy. "Where's the dog?" he asked.

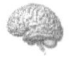

Christmas Eve, we went to Cathe and Tom's house again. Their daughter, Danielle, and her daughter, Michaela, were arriving from Houston to join the rest of the family. Would another holiday gathering provoke new oddness from Mike? After some shower protests, he understood we would walk to their house for dinner.

Once there, he smiled and seemed engaged to the extent possible. He sipped half a glass of Merlot and ate a small turkey sandwich. However, as soon as the sun went down, he picked up the dog and held her by the collar as if afraid he would lose her. He became agitated and started making angry faces at me and sharp motions at the door, indicating he wanted to leave. As he became more distraught and insistent, we said our goodbyes and prepared to head home. As we walked out the front door, Mike held the end of Bijou's leash, and while she was walking ahead of him, he turned to me with a frightened look and asked, "Where's the dog?"

Once back in our house, he turned on all the lights. I remembered a condition I had heard about called sundowners and googled it. Yes, some people with dementia undergo a change in emotions when it gets dark. They might experience sadness, anxiety, fear, agitation, restlessness, and irritability. Bingo! I then realized that he had been very sensitive to the darkening skies since the time change when fall began a couple of months ago. He would pull down the shades and turn all the lights on.

"We don't need every light in the house on," I had said irritably. I associated this with his boredom and the need to be doing something. What he was doing, I now realize, was closing the blinds on the coming darkness and shuttering out the night. I remembered the three occasions when we had recently been out after dark: Thanksgiving, a friend's early Christmas party, and now Christmas Eve at my sister's. All produced the same reaction. From now on, I resolved not to freak out about wasted electricity. I also thought that being away from his usual environment in the evening exacerbated the anxiety. I vowed to myself that in the future, we would plan to visit people before dark.

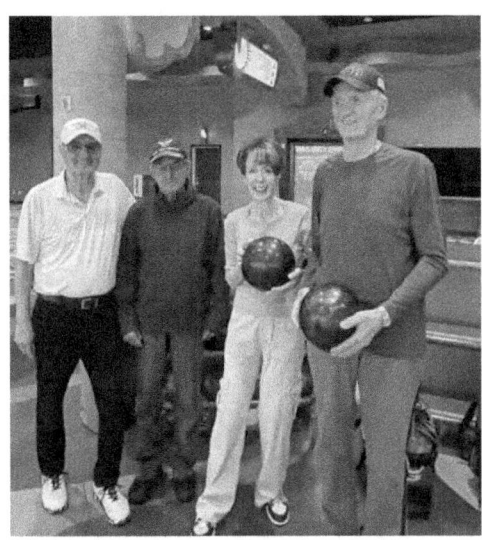

The Alley Ratz. Tom and John with Mike and me

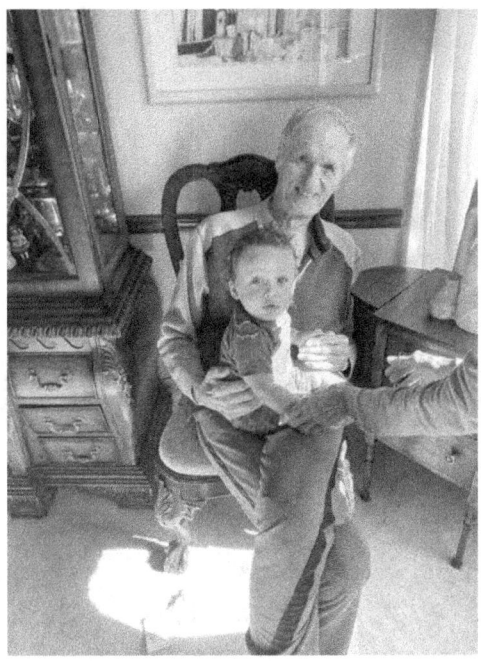

Mike and his great-grandson, Coa

Scene 29

2024: Six Years After Diagnosis—Sports and Entertainment

As the year began, and Ratt burrowed deeper into Mike's prefrontal cortex, I tried to fill his life with as many pleasurable activities as possible. I could still count on his interest in watching football, but only a few games were left before the Super Bowl and the season ended.

One might not understand how bleak life must have felt to Mike with so little to do. He couldn't read, write, or understand anything on TV. He couldn't enjoy a play, a movie, or games, listen to music, or visit with friends in person, on the phone, or social media. He couldn't ski, play golf or basketball, or do any other exercise besides walking. Going out to dinner or lunch was of little interest or pleasure. He couldn't even drive or bike anywhere.

The list of what he could no longer do was long and depressing. At least he had bowling and walks in the park with Bijou and me—for now. How could I help Mike have some quality of life and still have time to do what I wanted to do, like write, read, and work out? This became my biggest challenge.

With bowling three times a week, daily walks with the dog, preparing three meals a day, and getting both of us dressed, I had scant time to fit in writing and other chores I needed to do. At home, Mike was very considerate of my time spent writing on the computer, shopping, scheduling appointments, paying bills, and researching for this book. He would sit quietly in his chair and doze off for an hour or two, but understandably, he would become utterly bored after a while. He'd walk up and down the halls, murmuring and breathing loudly. This caused Bijou to come in and whine about something, and then I knew my time to accomplish anything was over. What brilliant idea did I have in my dwindling bag of tricks to engage and entertain these two?

On a Sunday evening in January, I invited Rick, whom we had met at bowling, to come over for dinner and watch an NFL playoff game with the KC Chiefs while his wife was out of town. He did not have the station it was to be broadcast on, but we did. He was delighted to accept, and Mike greeted him properly when he arrived. We all settled on the couch to watch the game.

After the first half, I paused the game for dinner. When we had finished eating, I cleared the dishes and then resumed the second half of the game. The dinner delay caused the game to go on until about 8:00. Around 7:00, Mike lost interest in the game and started staring daggers at me. Then he made quick, brushing motions with his hands, indicating that Rick should leave. Mike was ready for bed, and as far as he was concerned, Rick was overstaying his welcome.

Noticing Mike's irritation, Rick offered to leave, but I said sternly, "Mike, Rick will leave when the game ends. He's our guest." He settled down, and we watched the rest of the game. Rick then made a hasty retreat, and Mike went to bed. Ratt had trampled on all of his social graces.

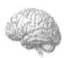

Super Bowl! I had been telling Mike all week that today was the big day. The Super Bowl was going to be played, and not only would it be here in Las Vegas, but the game was between the San Francisco 49ers and Patrick Mahomes and the Kansas City Chiefs—the Big Boys! An hour before game time, I reminded him again. No reaction.

At three thirty, I closed out the document that I had been working on—this book—came into the family room, turned on the game, and sat down on the couch beside him to watch. The first half was dull, and Mike showed no awareness that he was even watching it. Then, during the second half, the KC Chiefs came alive, the game got exciting, and it finally went into overtime. I gave a play-by-play, and Mike perked up. The Big Boys won! The bad news was that no more football would be televised until fall, seven long months away. I wondered, *Will he still be able to enjoy football next season?*

Football was over for the year, but bowling resumed, and we were back at the Sunset bowling lanes. Mike had, of course, been excited about the new bowling year. "We gotta get going. Win money!" he'd said over and over.

Part of the money we pay to bowl for league games goes into a fund. At the end of the season, the league distributes the money according to the team's ranking, and you can recoup some portion of what you'd paid out over the season. In both our Monday and Wednesday leagues, we ranked at the bottom, or near the bottom, for the last two seasons, and we had little hope of winning much money back for a few obvious reasons. Our team now resembled a "Who's on First" comedy routine.

Tom's brother had mental disabilities. He was stoic with no affect or emotion except for the occasional tight smile when he managed a strike. He walked with a wooden gait to the foul line, took seven or eight quick, unsteady steps, then hurled the ball in a gigantic arc to the left. The ball teetered dangerously on the right edge of the lane, then either rolled off into the gutter or miraculously hovered on the brink of disaster and hit the headpin for a strike. His game was erratic. Some days, he bowled forty pins above his average, and some days, twenty below.

We were also the last team to finish because he ritualistically used the restroom to wash his face and clean his glasses, prompting Tom or me to ask, "Where's John?" almost every time it was his turn to bowl. Then he'd sit at the table, eyes downcast, until Tom or I shouted, "You're up, John." At that point, he would come alive—well, he would jump up. "You're up, John," was our second most uttered phrase after "Where's John?" He was capable of bowling well, but it depended on his medication and mental state that day.

And then there was Mike, whose average had now slipped to 100. Adjusting his throw or stance for his second shot to aim at the remaining pins was beyond his capability. He used the same technique each time he threw the ball. Positioning himself on the far-left side of the lane, he took two steps to the right in a diagonal line, then hurled the ball on the far-right side with a powerful right-to-left twist of his wrist. Similar to John's technique, his ball rode the rail like a seasoned hobo, then either fell into the gutter or miraculously took a left turn and hit the headpin.

When he picked up the ball, I noticed Mike placed his left thumb in the thumb hole first, then pulled it out and put his right thumb and fingers into the holes. He needed occasional reminders that we threw two balls, not one, before he sat down again, so I stood behind him when he bowled to either direct him to his seat or back to the ball carrier for another hurl.

During the three games, I remained standing to announce whose turn it was to the players, like an air traffic controller on steroids. "You're up, John," or "Your turn, Mike." Jim, one of the other league players, called me the Den Mother. I had suggested to Tom that we change the team's name to the Dis-A-Bowls, but he rejected it. I think he thought it too politically incorrect.

Because Mike couldn't read the scoresheets, and partly because he did not seem to understand the whole team concept anymore, he assumed we were in first place, crushing the other teams. He only focused on his game. If he managed a spare or a strike once in a blue moon, he assumed he was bowling brilliantly, and we were winning. Mike thought we were leading in both leagues, and I encouraged this falsehood. It made him happy because he believed we were competing to win money—another falsehood I perpetrated. Without bowling, there would be little joy in his life, so I felt justified in my deceit.

Since Mike wanted to bowl every day, we joined a Friday practice group called the Alley Oops. When I let it slip that we were only practicing bowling with the Alley Oops group, he felt disappointed and didn't want to go, which initially seemed strange to me until I realized that it was about competing for points/money. "Win money. We need to bowl." Or his more common comment, "We need to get going! Win. Win money." To get him excited about bowling on Friday, I began to tell him that Friday's practice was also a league game, and when we finished, I told him we had won every game and got all the points. He was happy all the way home.

After a Wednesday league game one day this summer, I'd had a bad bowling day. I couldn't seem to pick up many spares, and I was cranky about it. As we left, Mike asked, as usual, "How'd we do?"

"Terrible," I grumbled truthfully for the first time. "We lost every game."

"Good. How many points?"

"Nothing! No points! We lost all three games," I shouted.

"That's great!" Mike said with a big smile.

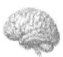

Mike's love of bowling taught me a valuable lesson. My friend Iris was going to a book signing for her book and asked me if I wanted to share a table with her. It was a Friday, the day we usually bowled with the Alley Oops group. I didn't have anyone to stay with Mike, so I'd planned to skip bowling since it wasn't a league game and take him to the book signing with me. I didn't think he'd know we'd be missing bowling and thought he would be happy to accompany me instead of being left home with a caregiver.

That morning, he was foggy. I tried to explain my plan and said that he needed to take a shower. He protested, as usual. "Why, where we going?" he whined. I told him again, quickly realizing that, of course, he did not understand. Or maybe he did and just didn't want to go.

"I want home in the chair with the dog," he sputtered. He was so sad and confused. Once again, I'd thought about this remarkable man I loved—a man who had so little in his life that gave him joy—and I decided to call my friend and beg off on the signing. *What did it matter that I might miss out on selling a few books?* I thought. I had so much to be grateful for, and he had so little.

When I decided to go bowling instead of to the book signing, I told Mike again that he needed to shower. He frowned and started to protest. "We're going bowling," I said, "so you need to shower." His face lit up, and he got up immediately and headed to the bathroom. I put his clean underwear, socks, and T-shirt on the bathroom vanity, reminded him to take out his hearing aids, turned on the shower to warm the water, and took out his dirty clothes to be washed as he shed them. I popped in twice to ensure he was using soap and shampoo, then let him alone to shower. When I heard the water stop, I waited a few minutes while he dried off, then put cream on the rash on his chest and handed him his hearing aids. I laid his clothes on his bed and then helped him dress.

After lunch, at 12:30, we drove to the Sunset for our two games with the Alley Oops group. Mike was, as usual, excited about the prospect of winning money. I eagerly agreed with him that we would win big. He was thrilled and engaged in life. What more could I ask?

Our standing "team" for Alley Oops was with Al, a man in his mid-80s who had painful arthritis and walked with a limp because of a past stroke. Still an excellent bowler, he walked up to the line slowly, stood still, then hurled the ball perfectly for a strike or spare. He proudly displayed the gold ring he'd been awarded for a perfect 300 game—pre-stroke. His wife, Twanna, also a good bowler, was ten years younger than he was. She was a sweetheart who occasionally brought their three-year-old autistic grandson to our practice. Ace sat quietly at the table with books and snacks. He also yelled, "Good job" after someone bowled and sometimes gave out high fives.

Recently, a new player named Peter and his stepdaughter–caregiver, Julie, joined us. Peter was ninety years old and had dementia as well. In his youth, he was a professional soccer player and was enthusiastic about bowling. We first put the side rails up, and he smiled and clapped, jumping up and down whenever he hit any pins. With a broad smile of surprise, his hands came up to his face and pressed against his cheeks in a gesture of amazement and happiness. It was so delightful watching his joy at his achievement. Mike also smiled, and I could tell he enjoyed having another disabled person struggling and succeeding to cheer on. Like Mike, his words could be mixed up. "You're a gambler!" Peter would exclaim happily when someone made a strike or a spare.

During the entire time—two games—Mike and Peter laughed, clapped, and gave each other high fives. In the middle of game two, Mike was ready to leave and go see the dog, but he persevered with my encouragement.

When we'd finished, I packed up the equipment and turned to notice that Mike had gone over to hug Peter and say goodbye to him. Julie and I looked at each other as the two said their goodbyes. They both smiled and vowed to return next week. All the other players on the Alley Oops team were effusive in their farewells to Mike. I was thrilled that I had changed plans for the day. It was indeed memorable. Before we left, we walked to the pro shop, and I had Mike's name engraved on the blue ball in fluorescent orange. Hopefully, it would be easier for him to find it in the rack when we bowled the following Monday.

I must say that bowling has been a real help in keeping our relationship close. Without it, there would be few things that we could still do together besides walking Bijou and the weekly dalliance in the bedroom. The blue straggler now struggled again, but innovation and flexibility were key to keeping our marital bond bound tightly.

On Wednesday, Mike asked me all morning to confirm that we were going bowling. We left at 12:30, right after lunch, for a 1:00 start time. He selected his lucky bowling cap from the large grouping he kept on the hall table and pointed at it. "Gonna win," he said with a confident smile, pointing at the hat. All the way there, in the car, he was Mr. Happy, chattering about killing the opponents.

"Yes," I intoned as usual. "We'll pulverize them, crush them, grind them into the ground." He laughed.

Mike had a bounce in his step as we walked in and retrieved the bowling balls from the locker. We located our lane and said hi to Tom, John, and fellow bowlers. Mike looked around, smiled, and whispered, "I can beat everyone."

"Yes, of course you can," I enthusiastically agreed. Although his average had now fallen to 85, the lowest in the league, Mike was happily oblivious.

At the end of the second game, with our team losing by over 150 pins, Mike motioned me to lean down. "Killing them," he confided with a conspiratorial smile.

"Yup," I whispered back.

With the game underway, Mike's jubilant mood continued. He made faces and did little dances and silly walks whenever he had managed a spare or a strike. He swooped his arms like a plane landing on a runway. Then he strutted to his seat, to which I directed him. Everyone around us laughed uproariously, unaccustomed to seeing him so animated.

"How'd we do?" he asked as he always had when we left and again several times on the way home.

"We did great," I said. "We won one game and got two points."

"That's good. Gonna win some money." He smiled. We are clinging to second-to-last place with one more game left to play in the season. Then he asked again, "Well?" His eyebrows arched in a quizzical gesture. "We got points?"

"Oh yeah," I continued, "killed 'em again."

"How many? Three?"

"Yup," I said, upping the lie. "All the points! Seven points." He held out his red hat and pointed at it with a big smile. "Lucky hat did it again!" I shouted.

When I kissed him good night that night, he said, "Bowl tomorrow?"

"No," I replied. "Bowl the next day."

"We'll think of something," he said with a happy look, and I felt momentarily sad because I knew there wouldn't be much fun for Mike tomorrow. He'll sit and look out the window.

He hugged and kissed me again, and I turned out the light by his bed and went into my bedroom to read. Soon, he popped in and waved. "Good night. I love you." I waved back and threw kisses, then followed him back to ensure he was tucked in. Every once in a while, this routine was repeated a few times before he finally went to sleep. After he was in bed, I had several hours to write and read, which I greatly enjoyed guilt-free.

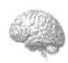

At the start of the year, during bowling league games, Mike knew that he followed me in the lineup and had few problems automatically getting up to bowl when it was his turn. A few months later, at the beginning of summer, I had to remind him when it was his turn to bowl. He also had trouble finding his seat afterward, sitting at the opponent's table or any nearby empty seat if I was not blocking and running interference. People smiled and waved me off when I rushed to relocate him, indicating they didn't care where he sat, but I smiled and guided him back to the correct table to take his seat.

By midsummer, I needed to lead him to the correct lane and help him find his ball. I turned it to where the finger holes showed, pointed at it, and then at the lane. I stood behind him when he bowled, reminding him to throw the second ball, and then directed him back to his seat. His bowling and, therefore, his scores were more erratic. When I moved ten or more steps away from him, he frantically looked around, unable to find me.

As spring rolled into summer, there was another change in Mike's bowling behavior. And this new development signaled to me, at least, that the damage had reached the prefrontal cortex of his brain. He had no patience for waiting anywhere longer than an hour and a half. The ability to delay gratification, manage impulses, and use mental processes to keep us from losing our cool or making rash decisions is a combination of key brain regions, with the prefrontal cortex—Mr. Big—being key. Control and patience rest here.[1]

Mike was now ready to leave after two games, and I had to coax him into playing the third one required in league bowling. I told him he didn't have to bowl—he could sit and watch—but he wanted the two of us to leave. "Where's the dog? Someone with her? Home alone?" he whined, pouting like a child told he couldn't have more cookies. Reluctantly, he bowled when it was his turn. "Last one?" he asked each time, a gloomy, angry look on his face.

On a Monday toward the end of summer, Mike had been anxiously awaiting bowling all weekend. The excitement was building. When we arrived at Sunset and saw the packed parking lot, he jokingly asked, "Why so many people here? They should be scared. We beat them." He laughed. Smiling, he was actually teasing about winning. Has Ratt not found the teasing neurons yet?

---

1. Neurolaunch.com.

"Yeah!" I played along as I always did. "We're going to crush them. Pulverize them. Grind them into the ground."

Midway through the second game, though, he looked at me and asked, "Done?"

"No. It's only the second game. We have to finish this one and play one more game." He made an angry face, pouted for the rest of the time, but got up and bowled when I prodded him.

When we had finally finished, and I told him he could put his regular shoes back on, he beamed. When we put away the bowling balls in the locker, he turned to me with a face full of expectation and asked, "Well, did we win?" Of course, I told him we did, and he beamed like a little leaguer whose team had finally won a game at the end of the season. His second question was, "When do we bowl again?" Then, of course, the inevitable, "Where's the dog?"

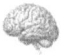

Football resumed in the fall of 2024, but as I had feared, Mike was uninterested in or unable to focus on even Kansas City Chiefs' football games. With football scratched from the entertainment list, bowling was now his only outlet and interest, and I worried that it, too, would end soon.

By early December, there weren't many days left for league bowling in the year because the league takes a two-week holiday break. Mike was excited to go bowling, as usual, and he kept up his good mood and jokes for the first two and a half games. He became a one-man comedy team, making faces, doing silly walks, and generally acting goofy after he bowled. The surrounding teams laughed good-naturedly at his antics, and he was encouraged to continue.

Then, in the middle of the third game, I looked at him and motioned that it was his turn to bowl. He stared at me gravely and shook his head.

Uh-oh, I thought. *He's hit the wall. His alarm clock just rang.* "Come on, Mike," I cheered, "five more to go. You can do it."

Others around us took up the chant, "Mike, Mike, Mike." He laughed and stood up. The two teams next to us began to smile, laugh, and encourage him. It was hilarious, and he was playing along, grinning and teasing. Then he smiled and happily bowled the last three frames, thrilled to be the center of attention and part of humanity.

By the end of the month, it became routine that he wanted to stop bowling after an hour and a half, and no amount of encouragement seemed to help. He got angry when I didn't leave, even though I'd told him he could sit there and watch, and we would go when I had finished the third game. But when I continued to bowl, his anger increased, and he stood up and walked behind our tables. I kept a close eye on him, and of course, minutes later, he looked around for me, anxiously, because he was disoriented. I guided him back to his seat, which he refused to sit in. I let him stand there as he glowered until I had finished playing.

By the end of 2024, whether we were bowling, visiting friends, or entertaining guests at home didn't matter. After an hour and a half, the alarm bells sounded, and he'd had enough—fini, kaput.

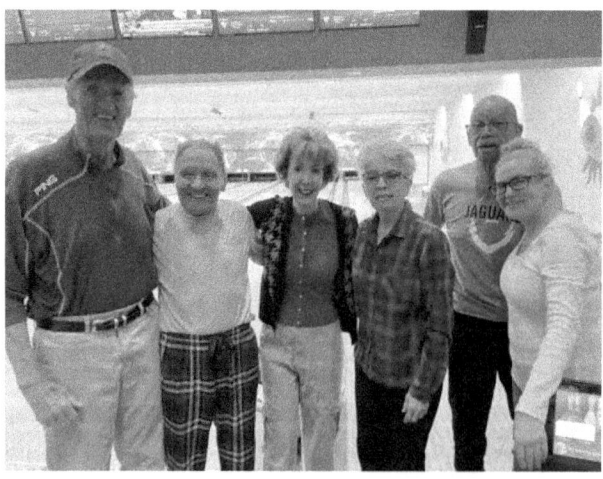

Our Alley Oops team: from left Mike, Peter, Sherry, Twanna, Al and Julie

Scene 30

Communicating with Man and Beast

Several times, beginning early in the year when I spoke to Mike, he had difficulty determining where my voice was coming from. If I sat in a chair to his left, reading a book, and asked, "Turn on TV?" he would turn to the right and repeatedly ask, "Where are you?" This became more frequent. The more I called out to him from the left, the more he turned to the right, unable to figure out the location of my voice. He could hear my voice with the benefit of his hearing aids, but he didn't understand what I said or from where the sound emanated.

The first thing Mike did in the morning was put in his hearing aids. His hearing aids are vital to him. Without them, he was almost entirely deaf. When the battery in his hearing aid went out, he urgently wanted help. Without being able to hear, he felt lost and panicky.

I was reminded that when Helen Keller, who had lost both her sight and hearing at nineteen months, was asked later as an adult if she could choose which sense she would have restored, she said she would choose to hear. "The problems of deafness are deeper and more complex, if not more important, than those of blindness. Deafness is a much worse misfortune," she'd said.

Hearing is a powerful sense that keeps us from isolation and allows us to connect with the world. But just hearing is not enough. We need to be able to understand what that sound that we hear is.

One day this year, after having replaced the battery in one hearing aid twice, I discovered it was not the battery that was dead. One of his hearing aids had failed, and he was distraught. I called the audiologist, and we quickly drove to her office, arriving fifteen minutes before closing. The device had indeed died but was still under warranty. Unfortunately, it had to be sent away for repairs, which usually took one to two weeks.

"Can we put a rush on it?" I had asked. "Mike keeps asking me to replace the battery because he cannot understand that the device is broken and needs to be repaired." After a quick call to the factory, the answer was yes, but there was a seventy-dollar charge. "Yes, please go ahead with the rush." A few days later, his hearing was restored.

A hearing aid helps us do just that—hear sounds. But understanding what those sounds mean takes a healthy brain. Is it a horn, a bark, a rustle in the trees, or a word? And if it's a word, what does the word mean? The auditory nerve runs from the cochlea in the inner ear to a station in the brain stem. Then neural impulses travel from that station up to the auditory cortex in the temporal lobe, where the brain attaches meaning to the sound that the ears have picked up.[1] The auditory cortex analyzes and decodes sound information by helping us recognize individual sounds and words. Mike's brain was damaged, so he could hear my words with the benefit of his hearing aid, but he struggled to locate the source of the sound and decipher what those words meant.[2]

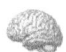

Besides Mike's inability to understand my words, his ability to speak words had vastly diminished over the six years since his diagnosis. I was aware, of course, that those with logopenic progressive aphasia slowly lose the ability to speak, write, read, and generally comprehend language, as LPA

---

1. Clevelandclinic.org.

2. practicalpie.com/practical psychology.

was first described as an impairment of language capabilities. At the same time, other mental functions were thought to remain intact. However, it is now recognized by experts that many—if not most—of those with LPA experience memory impairment, short-term memory formation, and loss of executive functions[3] in addition to the loss of language.

"Executive functions" is an umbrella term that includes a wide range of cognitive processes and behavioral competencies, including verbal reasoning, problem-solving, planning, sequencing, the ability to sustain attention, resistance to interference, utilization of feedback, multitasking, cognitive flexibility, and the ability to deal with novelty.[4] These are all controlled in the prefrontal cortex—Mr. Big—in the frontal lobe. Evolutionarily, this part of the human brain is the newest.

Conversations require the use of these higher thought processes, which Mike had mostly lost. Now, it's just straightforward communication. He tells me when he needs something. "Ears dead," he would say, pointing at an ear. This was his way of telling me that the battery in his hearing aid needed to be changed. By the way, he could have changed the battery by himself just a year ago, but now he cannot.

Mike made observations about the weather or buildings we had passed on the way to bowling, but most of those words were gibberish. *What* he was saying was not as important to me as the fact that he was trying to relate something, so I smiled and agreed with him. Sometimes, I expanded on the point I thought he was trying to make, although I knew he did not understand what I was saying back to him as it was now extremely difficult for him to understand language at all. However, he knew I was listening to him, which made him feel understood because he nodded and smiled.

---

3. National Aphasia Association.

4. Chan, R.C., D. Shum, T. Toulopoulou, E.Y. Chen. "Assessment of Executive Functions: Review of Instrumentsand Identification of Critical Issues." *Archives of Clinical Neuropsychology*. March 2008.

In some areas, Mike's brain worked fine. He could still understand danger. When Mike wanted my attention, he called, "Hey, hey, hey." While putting groceries away, I heard him shout, "Hey, hey, hey."

"What?" I answered in a tired, irritated voice.

"Look, look," he said, motioning to me. I followed him to the garage and discovered I had left the car running. In my defense, it's a hybrid, and it's keyless. If the door is not entirely closed, the engine won't turn off even though I've pressed the off button. And because it's so quiet, I can't hear the motor running when I step away.

"Thank you," I said and hugged him.

I often ponder his brain processes. He obviously thinks about things like my car running. I wondered how it was possible to think without words. For years, scientists believed we needed language to think, but apparently, that is not the case. We need language for higher thought, but several decades of research have shown that some people do not have an inner monologue, meaning they don't talk to themselves in their heads—they don't need words to think. Other research shows that people don't use the language regions of their brain when working on wordless logic problems, like sudoku. This is likely why he was able to do sudoku for so long. It involved numbers, not words.

Modern technologies, like functional magnetic resonance imaging (fMRI) and microscopy, give researchers an excellent picture of which parts of the human brain correspond to different functions. Neuroscientists have been able to approximate and map more specific functional regions associated with long-term memory, spatial reasoning, and speech.[5]

Of course, Bijou cannot speak or understand many words, either. Animals don't have language like humans, but they have their own

---

5. realclearscience.com/.

communication. When we walk past a secured wall and another dog is barking, she is not afraid and pays no attention. They must be barking something like, "I'd rip you to shreds if I could get out of the fenced yard," instead of, "Watch out! I'm coming to attack you." She understands their intent.

Although their language may not be as highly evolved as ours, according to National Geographic, "Life is very vivid for animals. In many cases, they know who they are. They know who their friends are and who their rivals are. They have ambitions for higher status. They compete. Their lives follow the arc of a career, like ours do. We both try to stay alive, get food and shelter, and raise some young for the next generation. Animals are no different from us in that regard."[6] I learned that dogs also have a prefrontal cortex, where "executive functions" are located—Mr. Middle Manager? Of course, the prefrontal cortex is more highly developed in humans. It makes up 10 percent of a dog's brain compared to one-third of a human's.[7]

Mike and Bijou communicate similarly. Neither can understand complicated sentences, but both attempt to communicate their needs and wants. Bijou and I communicate much like Mike and I do. When I explain something to her in long, complicated sentences like, "We're going bowling, Bijou, we'll be back later. Don't worry," she just stares at me and cocks her head. I'm sure she heard, "Blah blah blah, later." When she barks, attempting to communicate something to me, there are different tones I can recognize. A loud bark, where the barks are close together, means someone or something, like a car, is out in front of the house. If the barking gets louder and more rapid, someone is approaching the front door. Short, piercing barks or a whine mean she wants a walk or food. Rhythmical barks about three seconds apart tell me Mike has trapped her in the bathroom.

---

6. nationalgeographic.com.

7. firstvet.com. "Everything You Need to Know About Your Dog's Brain."

This rhymical bark is a call. She uses it if she wants to go in or out of the front door, where she does not have access to a doggie door. She also employs it when she is caught in the garage after Mike and I have entered the house, and I had assumed that she ran in first. These calls from the garage are, of course, muffled but very distinct and urgent.

Without the ability to converse, Mike and I grunt and point like dogs or monkeys, stopping just short of picking lice out of each other's hair. "Look, a child. Watch out, car." But like Bijou, Mike and I can't discuss how we feel or our thoughts on the current state of affairs with any specificity because the part of his brain required for higher thought is damaged in his brain.

Like Bijou, if I use a complete sentence without pantomime to Mike, he can't understand what I am saying, either. Perhaps my words sound to him like, "Blah, blah, blah, dinner." Or "Blah blah blah, bowling." When he speaks to me, I, in turn, hear, "Ball sky bringle frap cloud high high nurpe wet." I watch his face. If he points at the sky, I realize he is trying to say something about the fact that it has stopped raining or there is a plane flying overhead. A lot of guesswork is involved in communicating with both Mike and Bijou. "Yes, it's nice and sunny today," I say, nodding. He smiles. He probably heard, "Blah, blah, blah, sunny."

I use pantomime and sign language with Bijou now as well because, ironically, she seems to also be losing her hearing, and she doesn't have the benefit of hearing aids. But she understands sign language. Waving my hand back and forth means no more treats or no walk now. Pointing my finger in the direction of her food bowl several times, she understands, then saunters slowly toward it. She doesn't hear the ringtone at the front door any longer or hear us returning home, running to greet us. I startle her when I bend to pet her, awakening her. She didn't know we had come home.

The Fourth of July passed without any angst on her part. In years past, she would have cowered for two days wrapped around the toilet bowl, wearing her Thunder Jacket, headphones with doggie music, and medicated with relaxers. This year, she barely stirred. I also think some of her odd behaviors, like covering her food, may be signs of senility—doggy dementia. The vet agrees that it's entirely possible. Another one of life's great ironies.

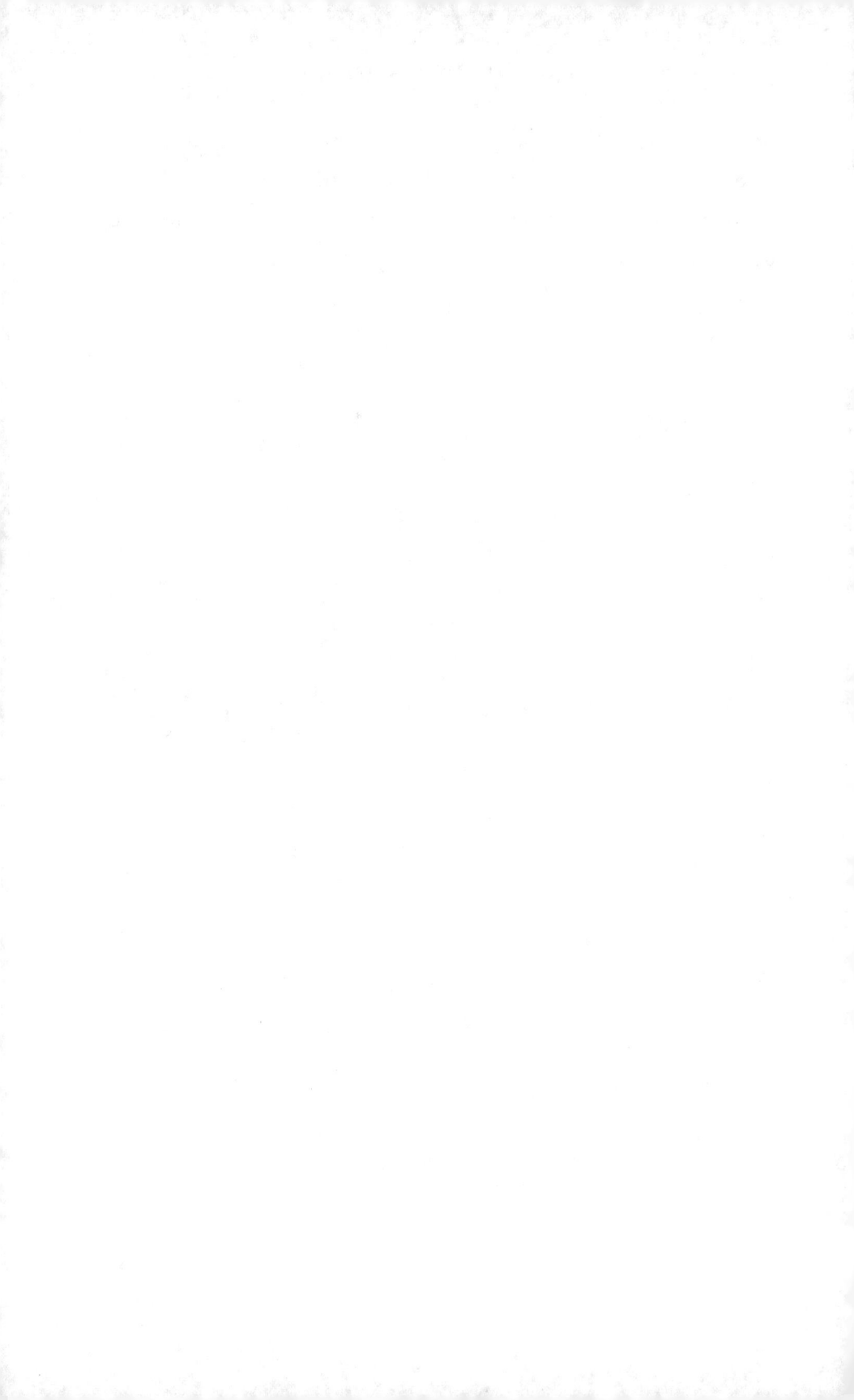

Scene 31

Losing Agency

Mike is, of course, totally dependent on me at this point. He has lost his agency—the psychological concept that includes forethought, implementation, self-management, learning, and adapting. He has lost most language and cannot complete a sentence with more than two or three words. His phrases have few nouns because he does not remember what many objects are called. He tries to speak, but his words are garbled and unintelligible. Sometimes, he realizes this and stops trying. At other times, he murmurs to himself in a low tone.

He can no longer go anywhere alone and would not know how to get there if he could. He doesn't know what day it is, and even though he looks at his watch frequently, he cannot tell the time. Since he's unable to use a phone or computer, he would be utterly lost outside. He couldn't even call 911 in an emergency. He understands this dependency and is careful not to stray too far from me. It is also why he is so fearful when I leave him with another caregiver.

For my part, I realize this is a lot of power to have over someone else's life, and I tread lightly so that he doesn't feel railroaded or manipulated. He is an adult, not a child, and he needs to feel as though he has some control over his life. Sometimes that takes great patience on my part, and I am not, by nature, a patient person.

Here are several examples. At the beginning of 2024, I watched Mike sit in his La-Z-Boy chair most of the day, wearing his golf shirts, slacks, leather belt, and shoes. He looked uncomfortable for just relaxing at home. First,

I assumed he would prefer slippers to shoes, so I bought him sheepskin slippers from Hammacher Schlemmer. They were soft and closed with a large Velcro strap, which I thought would be easy for him to put on and wear.

After a few days of indulging me, he pushed back, saying he liked wearing his shoes in the house. This was a Miranda day. I was preparing breakfast, and again, I was rushing to get him dressed and me ready to leave when she arrived. I walked over to him, raised my voice, and said, "Great, I showed you the slippers online before I ordered them, and you approved. You don't need to wear your shoes in the house when you are just sitting in your chair all day."

He couldn't understand the words I was spewing, but he knew I was unhappy because he didn't want to wear the slippers. He looked sheepish and sad, and tears filled his eyes. "W-w-why, why do you?" he stammered. I knew immediately that he was trying to say, "Why do you care or have a say in what I want to wear?"

I huffed around the kitchen for a few minutes and asked myself that exact question. *Why is it so important that I get my way?* He has so little control over his life. It was my turn to look sheepish. I approached him, kissed him on the forehead, and said, "You wear whatever you want, honey." Responding to the contrite gesture, more so than my words, his lips parted in a small smile. He happily, though I imagine pretty uncomfortably, wore his slacks, belt, and shoes daily in the house—at least for the next few months. However, he won this round, exerting some measure of control over his life.

He definitely needed a new belt. *This should be an easy one,* I thought. Mike had lost a lot of weight. Five years ago, he weighed 205 pounds; in 2024, he was down to 165 pounds. His old belt is size 38, and he showed me it was too big. I went online and ordered a similar one, size 34. He put it on when it arrived and pronounced it, "Good." The following few days, he refused to wear it. It immediately became an alien belt that he neither recognized nor liked. I sent it back.

Next, I bought him two pairs of athletic pants—joggers—online. I showed them to him on the website, and of course, he said, "Good." I thought they would be easier for him to put on and much more comfortable wearing them in the house. One pair is black and one is gray, with a white stripe down the sides. They are typical, loose-fitting, nylon gym pants, the kind he has worn over basketball shorts for years.

In the morning, when I started to help him put the sweatpants on, he got upset. "I don't like these," he protested. "They're ugly." After several unsuccessful attempts to get him to wear them over the next few days, I gave up and put them away in his closet. He pulled on his slacks and cinched up the too-big leather belt that hung a foot from his waist. He smiled broadly, testing my vow to let him wear what he wanted. And so, the athletic pants hung in the closet, unworn.

Four months later, he emerged from his bedroom one afternoon wearing said pants. "Look," he proclaimed proudly, as if he'd discovered that Nike had planted a tree of athletic wear in his closet. "Look! New. These are great."

"Yes," I said, shocked. "They look great on you and must be so comfortable. You have two pairs, one black and one gray. Here is the other one." He smiled like a kid with a new toy. I once again mentally slapped my forehead. Once he began wearing the joggers, he refused to wear the slacks at all. At least the belt problem was solved, and he was in control.

I tried once more. In May, it began to get hot. The temperatures were in the nineties, so I pulled out Mike's cargo shorts from last year. We tried them on, and they were too big because he had lost so much weight. We drove to Dillard's, and in the men's department, he tried on Polo-brand shorts without pockets because he now thought the casual cargo shorts he had worn and preferred for years were "ugly." He tried the new shorts on, declared they were good, so we paid for them and took them home.

The following day, when I had placed the shorts on his bed for him to wear, he looked at them as though they were covered in dog do. "No!" he shouted, wrinkling his nose. Then he pulled out his new favorite athletic pants and put them on. My forehead is permanently dented from all the head slaps. The two pairs of golf shorts sat unworn in his closet for the entire summer. I would have returned them, except I kept hoping he would rediscover them like he had the athletic pants and decide that they would become his new favorite items of clothing. However, as I write these words almost a year later, they still hang in his closet. Maybe next summer?

I took Mike with me one day this summer when I got my hair cut and colored. Patti cut Mike's hair while my roots were being magically transformed from gray to brown. This entire ordeal lasted two hours, and he was unhappy about sitting in the chair, watching while I was beautified. I would think that it would be more interesting than staring at a TV, but he pouted.

Since we were there at noon, I packed lunches for us. I put his peanut butter and jelly sandwich, raisins, and chocolate chip cookies on a plate and set them on the table beside him. "Eat your sandwich," I said calmly. He didn't move. "Eat. See, I'm eating mine." He remained still. "Mike, eat!" He slowly shook his head, indicating no. He had lost so much weight and rarely finished a meal. "Eat!" I commanded. He again stubbornly shook his head back and forth.

He was so defiant, I wanted to push his face into the sandwich and stomp on the cookie. Instead, I took a deep breath and reminded myself I was a mature adult. Mr. Big worked well in my brain. It was Mike who had so little control over anything in his life. I told him when to dress, shower, and eat. This was one thing he could control. I couldn't force-feed him, so he had taken a stand and refused to eat there in the beauty shop on principle.

"Okay, fine," I said, taking several more deep breaths. I wrapped the sandwich back up and put it away. When we got home, I unwrapped it and put it on a plate at the table where he usually eats. "Your lunch is ready," I said casually, and he walked over, sat down, opened his Diet Coke, and began eating. Mike four, Sherry zero.

Of course, he has no control over where I take him. In July, I needed to visit a girlfriend, a fellow writer, who was helping me with my website. It was Saturday, and after taking the dog to the park, we headed a half hour north to her home. I had told him several times of my plans, of course, but he did not understand.

"Where we going?" he asked in that whiney tone accompanied by the *I smell something nasty* nose wrinkle.

"To my friend's house. She's helping me."

Thirty seconds later, "Where we going?"

"To my friend's house. She's helping me." This went on for the next twenty minutes, and I reminded myself why it had been an excellent decision not to drive to California to see our grandsons and new great-grandson last November. Four hours of "Where we going?" and I would want to strangle him—compassionately and lovingly, of course, but strangle him nonetheless.

Mike doesn't like going to unfamiliar places because he doesn't know where he is, and I imagine that is disorienting. But he does not want to stay alone for any length of time now. So I knew he would want to ride with me on a small errand I needed to make at the bank, but I went through the routine of giving him some decision-making control. "I have to go to the bank to deposit a check. Do you want to go or stay here?" I asked him.

"What?"

Then I remembered that offering choices didn't work anymore. I slowly repeated, "I am going to go to the bank. Do you want to come?"

"What? Where you going?"

"To the bank. Do you want to come?"

"Where you going?"

"To the bank." I changed the question. "Do you want to stay here with Bijou?" That he understood.

"*I'll* go with you," he said brightly, jumping up as if I had asked for a volunteer to step forward.

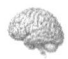

Mike's frustrations in losing control of his life are sometimes quite evident. He is usually angry when I hand him his toothbrush at bedtime. "I just did that," he yells.

"I know, but we have to do it every night. I'm going to go brush mine now," I answered, leaving him to brush. I peeked around the corner, ensuring the toothpaste was still on the brush and the brush was in his mouth.

When I told him today was shower day, he resisted, as usual. Our shower is a glass enclosure with a bench-type seat at one end, one-inch tile on the floor, and a grab bar on the wall. Until today, I would turn on the water, help him undress, and direct him into the tiled pen. I could then leave the bathroom, knowing he would stand under the showerhead and generously apply the body wash/shampoo, lathering his body and hair. I knew this because I would peek into the bathroom to make sure it was being done.

Today, however, I was in a hurry and impatient. When I finally got him to step into the shower enclosure, he was furious and didn't want to put his head under the showerhead to wash his hair. "What you doing?" he screamed as I gently tried to guide his head under the water from outside the shower. He is a good foot taller than I am, so this was not an easy feat.

I was afraid that he would angrily slam the shower door closed to thwart me and amputate my arm, so I backed out of the shower.

"Wet your head," I directed, pointing at my head and standing a safe distance from the shower.

He has always washed his hair automatically, if not willingly. This time, he did not seem to understand that he needed to wet and soap his hair. *Did he not understand, or was he trying to exert some control?* I finally sneaked in behind him and stuck a glob of shampoo on his head, and with him screaming, he and I finally got it rinsed off. I was soaked by the time the shower session ended, and I looked like a cat that had fallen into a pond—physically soaked and mentally drained.

As I helped him get dressed, I reviewed my options for the future. If this was where he was, enduring a dramatic and harrowing shower scene three times a week would not work. Changing the showerhead to one with a long, handheld attachment seemed like a no-brainer, but not the entire answer. Showering him would only work if he was compliant and sat quietly on the bench like a capybara—which I'd read were extraordinarily docile and chill giant rodents—while I hosed him off. At best, this option seemed awkward.

Then I thought of showering with him, but I didn't want to get into a brawl in a wet shower with glass doors while we were naked. Next, I considered an aide who could come to the house, but I quickly nixed that. If he resisted me, he would definitely not want some stranger wrestling him into submission. Finally, I settled on option three—ordering adult bath wipes and dry shampoo for the time being and foregoing the shower, except maybe once a week.

We are both type A personalities, which served us both well as leaders and managers. In our marriage, however, I tended to defer to him, partly because of my generational mantra that the husband should lead, and partly because I looked up to him so much. Now, I am in charge and need to tamp down my instinct to take control. My supposedly mature, functioning human brain knew that when Mike defied my entreaties to shower or take medicine, it was dementia, not him. However, my reptilian brain wanted to scream and pound him into submission. Screaming did sometimes make me feel better, and I allowed myself this guilty pleasure once in a while in the privacy of my home. ARRRRGGGG!

The showering supplies arrived, but of course, he has taken a shower without complications or major complaints ever since. He is compliant as long as we are going bowling, and I am playful, not pushy. Another lesson.

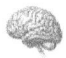

Even though he was now unable to have an orgasm, the ultimate pleasure and release during sex, just the act itself and the human connection seemed to suffice for Mike until mid-2024. Then it became difficult for him to even get an erection with Viagra, and he blamed the pills. "These old. Need new ones," he said angrily. I knew the pills had not expired and that the real problem was the sex organ between his ears, not the one between his legs. Each week, I continued giving him the blue pill and leading him into the bedroom, but he became more and more hesitant, exclaiming, "It doesn't work," pointing at his penis.

"That's okay," I said. "Let's just try." He protested the last couple of times I tried to coax him into bed, reluctant to fail again and with no apparent interest in trying. On Sunday, our date morning, he sat in his living room chair. I handed him the blue pill and a glass of water and raised my eyebrows seductively. He looked at me and frowned.

"Just take it," I said, "and we'll go cuddle for about a half hour, then see what happens." I smiled what I thought was an alluring smile.

"No good," he said, shaking his head.

"Just take it, and we'll try."

He looked at me, shook his head, and smiled sadly. "No more," he said with finality. *Was that the end of our sex life?* I wondered. Besides his physical inability to orgasm, had Ratt severed his sexual desire neurons?

Using fMRI, scientists have pinpointed several regions of the brain that kick in when people feel sexual desire. As suspected, several of them are in the temporal lobe, one of the damaged lobes in Mike's brain. One of those regions, the amygdala, orchestrates powerful emotions. Another, the hippocampus, manages our memories. It may become active as we associate sights and smells with past sexual experiences. Had Mike lost those sweet memories and, therefore, any sexual desire?

Scene 32

Expect the Unexpected

This year, Mike occasionally exhibited strange behaviors that occurred randomly, not regularly. We have a doggie door for Bijou, and she uses it to go into the walled, gated backyard as the mood or nature moves her, as she has for thirteen years. As I was preparing dinner one evening, early in the year, Mike suddenly screamed, "Where's Bijou?" as if he had just learned dognappers were skulking around in the neighborhood, and she needed to be located immediately.

Startled, I pointed and said, "She's outside in the backyard." His jaw dropped, and his mouth hung open in utter disbelief. It was as if I had said that I sold her to the local kill shelter. "It's okay," I soothed, surprised. "She's fine." At that moment, Bijou pushed open the doggie door and entered the house, totally oblivious to the drama unfolding. Mike lunged for her and grabbed her collar, holding her to prevent her from going out again. Bijou had a look on her face that said, "What the @#%**&^& is going on?"

"Put her down, Mike, she's fine," I prompted. And reluctantly, he did. It was several months before he repeated that odd behavior. In the past, I would immediately worry that any unusual behavior on his part was the start of a downhill slide. I realize now that he may do something new one day and not the next. With dementia, the new behavior can be a one-off. It does not necessarily constitute the beginning of a new pattern.

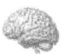

One afternoon in the spring, I'd decided to water the newly planted rosebush in the front yard. I walked out the front door, leaving it open. When I finished, only a few minutes later, I tried to go back into the house but discovered that Mike had locked both the security and front doors. I rang the doorbell several times and banged on the side panel, a stained-glass window, in an attempt to get his attention. As I cupped my hands around my eyes and pressed my nose to the glass, I saw Mike sitting in his easy chair. Bijou was frantically jumping and barking. Knowing I had locked the interior garage door, I rang the front doorbell twice again.

Finally, I saw Mike get up and walk toward the door. Thank goodness, I thought. It's ninety-five degrees out here. But instead of coming to the door, he walked to the front of the room and stared at me through the picture window. I was clearly visible, flapping my arms up and down like a bird preparing for takeoff, gesturing for him to unlock the door. He stared, nodded at me, then walked back and sat down in his chair.

I rang again and pounded on the door. Again, he got up and went to the front window. My face, now dripping with sweat, was inches from his. "Open the freaking door!" I yelled. I was now jumping up and down, pointing at the front door and making turning motions with my hands. He nodded, smiled, and then went and sat back down in his chair. Fortunately, I remembered I had a key hidden in the backyard, so I retrieved it and let myself in. Then I plopped down on the couch, hot and exhausted. I'm sure the neighbors think that I'm a lunatic.

I now have hidden keys in both the front and back yards and carry a set when I walk down to the mailbox only twenty yards away, as Mike is quick to close and lock any open doors he sees. I had an iron fence installed around our front yard so that Bijou could have more outdoor space, but I need to teach her how to unlock the front door because I frequently hear muffled barks and discover that she, too, has been shut out of the house. He is oblivious to this. Even when he could clearly—I assume—see us, it didn't occur to him that he was locking us out of the house.

This year, Mike no longer remembered to walk Bijou in the morning. He had quite forgotten that he ever did, and she was now at an age where she enjoyed sleeping in. I continued the ritual of daily afternoon walks with the three of us.

One afternoon in the summer, I grabbed Bijou's harness and leash and got them both into the car to take them to Fox Ridge Park, where we walked the quarter mile under the trees. Halfway around the track, a large, white dog—part husky, part devil—raced toward Bijou, grabbed her by the head, and pinned her to the ground. As the panic-stricken owner, I tried to pull the dog off Bijou, the squeals and sounds of pain and terror from our precious dog bloodcurdling. I would have thought that Mike would have been apoplectic, but he stood there calmly, staring as if he were watching a movie, apparently not understanding what was happening. Afterward, as I was frantically driving to the vet, he calmly asked, "Was it a child?"

"Was what a child? No, a dog attacked Bijou." It was as if he couldn't comprehend what he had clearly just witnessed. He silently and calmly began petting her. It certainly wasn't the reaction I would have expected, but I was glad he was not upset.

Bijou was fine after they sedated her and stitched up a gash in her neck. Days later, she happily returned to the park but was cautiously on the lookout for potential attackers. And I carried a stun gun that I had hastily ordered on Amazon.

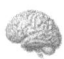

On Monday, we had again headed to the park after bowling and lunch. It was still 110 degrees, but under the shade of the trees, it felt like only 100.

Since Cathe and Tom were out of town, we stopped by their house to pick up their dog, Gobi.

As usual, Mike gripped Bijou's leash at the park, and I took Gobi's. After a few minutes, Gobi squatted to do her business, and I reached for a doggie do-do bag to retrieve the poop. Picking it up, I realized there was a hole in the bag, and I ended up with most of it on my hands.

Mike stared at my hands, very alarmed. "What happened?" He screamed as if I were covered in blood.

"Nothing. I got poop on my hands."

"What? What did you do?" he shouted again for the third time.

"Nothing. The bag was broken." I pointed at the restroom. "I'm going into the bathroom to wash my hands."

"My God!" he roared. "You've got to stop this shit."

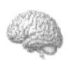

One of our evening standbys had been music videos of bands and performers from our era, played at a moderate volume. One night this summer, I clicked on Freddy Mercury and Queen singing "Bohemian Rhapsody."

"Noooo!" Mike yelled, flapping his arms like an angry aircraft marshaller directing a plane to the runway. "No! He's dead!" So much for Freddie Mercury. I tried Elvis. These were two regulars he had enjoyed as recently as last week. "NO!" he said again with a grimace that looked as though he had just eaten rotten eggs. "He died!" I switched to Bruno Mars and "Uptown Funk."

"Still here?" he asked me.

"Yes, he performs here in Vegas."

"Good," he said, settling in to watch the video for at least the 110th time.

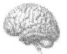

By the end of summer, Mike was ready for bed before 7:30. There was nothing he could watch on TV anymore except a few *America's* or *Britain's Got Talent* videos, and he couldn't focus on them for long. He declared all the singers terrible and was unimpressed with everyone else.

At 7:15, I turned the TV off one evening and set the security alarm. Mike checked the window shades, which he had pulled down hours ago. Then suddenly, he walked to the coffee table and looked down, pointing at Bijou, who was lying under it, fast asleep. "Right here! Right here! Right here!" he shouted, as if she had been missing for weeks and somehow managed to crawl home through raging fires and attacking animals to drag herself into the house and collapse under the coffee table, exhausted.

"Thank God you found her," I told him. "I've been worried sick."

Of course, all of these behaviors were both strange and amusing, but how to explain them? What was going on in his brain? Who knows? Certainly not Bijou or me.

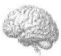

In the fall, because Mike began going to bed even earlier, at about 7:00, he got up earlier and entertained me with dances when he emerged from his bedroom. Each morning, after I had been reading the paper for a half hour, he sashayed into the living room doing a silly walk or pantomimed Steve Martin doing King Tut.

Since he slept in his socks, briefs, and T-shirt, he only needed to pull on his athletic pants and slip into his shoes to dress initially, which he could still do without help. He rubbed his chin, showing me he had shaved. "All done," he said proudly each morning, and then he duck-walked, Charlie Chaplin style, over to the picture window to sit in the dining room chair.

He turned back several times to ensure I was laughing uproariously, and of course, I guffawed and told him, "You're a goofy guy," which delighted him. Then I finished the paper and made breakfast.

This morning, I went into his bedroom before he emerged. He was standing by his bed, wearing his T-shirt and underwear. "Good morning," I chirped. He looked at me, squinted his eyes, and, with a smirk, turned around, lowered his undershorts, and mooned me.

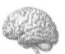

His behaviors could be strange, endearing, and delightful. I was preparing dinner one evening. Mike sat down at the kitchen table, and I gazed at this still-handsome man who had given me such pleasure and love over the past fifty-plus years. He smiled, and I felt overcome with emotion at how cheerfully he tried to navigate his increasingly incomprehensible world with smiles and laughs, playfully trying to make me laugh, trying to connect.

"Look, look, come here, Sherry," he said, pointing out the window, his face as amazed as a toddler's. "Clouds," he sang out. I wanted to finish what I was doing, but I joined him at the window.

"They're beautiful," I said, "and it doesn't look like rain." After a few minutes, I kissed him and returned to making dinner. I reminded myself that he was connecting, which is more important than having dinner ready a few minutes later than planned.

I marveled at the small things he managed to find joy and pleasure in, so guileless—the sun moving from behind the clouds to warm our faces, the laughter of little children at the park, the dog rolling in the grass, a full moon. Of course, anytime Mike thought about bowling, he smiled and repeated his mantra. "We've got to get going!" he'd say out of nowhere in a commanding voice. "We need points. Get money." Gazing up at the clouds, he gestured to the patches of blue sky. He did silly dances. At these moments in time, he is alive. He had few thoughts about the past and none of the future, at least as far as I could tell.

Scene 33

2024: Balancing Life on a High Wire

One Saturday, around the first of the year, my brother, Derreck, stopped by, and we chatted and got caught up with recent life events. Mike was sitting in his chair, unengaged in the conversation. After checking with Derreck, I said to them both, "I have a nail appointment. I'll be back in a half hour." I kissed Mike goodbye.

Thirty minutes later, I texted Derreck to tell him I would be a bit late as the manicurist was running behind and I would return at 5:30, an hour after I had left. Derreck called me en route to say that Mike was agitated and wanted to know when I would be back. It was getting dark, and it was his dinnertime. I said that I was five minutes away.

When I walked in, Mike gave me an angry face and said sarcastically, "Thanks!! You, you."

This totally annoyed me. He was with my brother, whom he had known since we were nineteen. I looked at him and said, "What?" I was furious. I had been gone for one hour. "You have no right to be angry at me," I said. I am with Mike almost constantly. I know he cannot understand that, but how do I respond? Do I let it go, try to explain, or show him an angry face? This time, I chose the latter.

"You have no right to be angry at me," I said again, giving him a furious face back. "I am angry at you!" This made me feel better, but I don't know what it meant to him. Once again, he sees I am out free, and his own brain imprisons him. As usual, he is over his anger quickly. It took me a couple of minutes longer.

Again, I had thought about dispensing with caregivers, both paid and related. Mike can sit with me while I get my nails done. Then I thought about grocery shopping. Mike pushes the cart, but it takes me twice as long to shop. If he insists on bringing Bijou, it's a half-day endeavor. I now draw the line at grocery shopping with Mike and Bijou. First of all, she hates going. The crowds, the chaos, and the clattering carts scare her.

Initially, I set her in the front of the cart, shortened the leash, and petted her to keep her calm. A grocery store employee informed me it was permissible to bring the dog, but they specified she could not ride in the cart for Health Department reasons and must be walked on a leash. Mike wanted to push the cart and hold Bijou's leash. Trying to direct the cart and guide Mike and Bijou around other customers to avoid tripping them with the leash while selecting groceries is stressful and not very artful. We must have looked like a clumsy Cirque du Soleil act without the costuming or music.

It took twice as long to shop, and I ended up exhausted. I am also sure other shoppers and employees wondered why I took this circus on the road. I now leave Bijou at home, which means two trips in the car—one to take them to the park and bring Bijou home, then the second excursion to the grocery store. There must be a better solution.

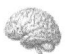

Miranda had been "adult sitting" with Mike for a year now. I had thought that over time, he would realize that I was coming back and that he could ignore her presence as he sat in his armchair, stared at the TV, and waited for me. However, his anger at her seemed to have increased instead of decreased, and it was always stressful for me to leave him with her.

As usual, when I pulled into the garage at 2:00 after having been gone three hours, he opened the back door and glared at me, his jaw set in an angry grimace. If he were a cartoon character, fumes of smoke would have been coming from both sides of his mouth.

We said goodbye to Miranda, and he sat down hard in his chair. In a slow, deliberate tone, he said, "I ... don't ... like ... her." He had said this a few times before, and I'd asked him why, but of course, he couldn't express himself fully. I know she is not physically abusive. She fixes his lunch, and the rest of the time, she is, I assumed—as she had been several times when I popped in through the garage door unannounced—on the phone. Since there was little interaction, I wondered why he was so resentful toward her.

I thought of the many conversations she and I have had upon my return or before I leave. She talked at you instead of with you. She is very opinionated, dismisses his condition, and doesn't appear to be at all empathetic. When I shared a funny story about something Mike had said or done, she always replied flippantly, "Oh, they are all like that," sweeping every person with dementia into this cubbyhole of behavior.

I thought, *No, they are not all like that. They are unique individuals with damage to various parts of their brains.* Still, I didn't understand how her presence bothered him. He sat in his chair when I was at home and on the computer in the other room. What difference does it make to him who is in the house?

"What don't you like?" I pressed him again.

"She is mean. She's not my friend. She just wants money." He articulated this clearly. I have never told him she gets paid to stay with him, but he is not stupid.

"Okay," I told him. "I will find somebody else."

"Oh, thank you," he said, relief pouring out of him. "Thank you."

I called the agency and spoke to the manager. I explained to her that I had no complaints about Miranda. "She shows up on time and prepares his lunch, but Mike said that he doesn't like her. I don't know if he means her in particular or if he means anyone replacing me. Given Mike's particular dementia, it is, of course, difficult to understand what exactly is bothering him," I explained. "However, I don't know for sure, and I don't want to discount his feelings. There may be an actual personality conflict. I want someone else to come out and see how he reacts." She said she understood and would let Miranda know we were taking a break for a while.

"No one needs to come this Thursday while you look for a suitable candidate," I said.

"What kind of person do you think would be a good fit?" she asked.

"Given Mike's inability to communicate easily, there is not much the person can do to interact with him. He can't play even simple games and cannot follow much on TV, so I'm not sure. But certainly, a kind person with a lot of empathy." And I added, "It would help to be a dog lover. Mike cherishes his Bijou." Love me, love my dog. I noticed that Miranda had never petted Bijou in greeting, even though the dog jumped excitedly when she came in. Instead, she just offered her hand for her to sniff.

On Friday, the manager from the Home Instead agency called me back to say they had a candidate who might be a good fit. Her name was Nancy, and we agreed she should come next Tuesday to see Mike's reaction.

On Tuesday, at precisely 11:00 a.m., a car pulled up in front, and a pleasant-looking woman in her late sixties, her gray hair pulled back in a ponytail, walked up to the house. She wore a nurse's smock, sensible shoes, and no discernible makeup.

I opened the door and greeted her warmly, introducing myself. She was, of course, Nancy. I invited her in and introduced her to Mike. I showed her around the house, and we sat and chatted about her background. She used to be in sales and has been a widow for the past six years with two adult children. She told me she had been with the agency for eight years.

I showed her what Mike ate for lunch, where it was located, how the TV controller worked, and what he watched on YouTube. I explained the Frameo electronic frame with pictures that I suggested she ask him about while they were eating lunch, and then I pointed out the dozen-plus picture books of our past travels that they could leaf through together. After half an hour, I kissed Mike and said I was off to the gym.

At 2:00, I pulled into the garage, fully expecting to see Mike's head poking out of the garage door leading to the house, his angry face showing his displeasure at being left behind. However, he was not there, and as I cautiously opened the door, I saw that not even Bijou had come to greet me.

As I walked into the family room, the three of them were sitting on the couch, and Mike was laughing. When he saw me, he smiled and made brushing motions with both hands, indicating that I could leave. Astounding. They were having fun! Nancy told me they paged through the vacation books, watched some videos, and "talked" the entire time. Mike appeared thrilled to have someone who had spent so much time and attention on him. He is not a vegetable. He's a real human being with thoughts and feelings. I didn't know whether to cry, jump for joy, or hug Nancy, so I did all three.

Two days later, Nan returned. Mike smiled when he saw her. At 2:00, when I'd arrived back home, I opened the garage door and walked in. Once again, they were happily "engaged," laughing and watching a women's bowling tournament. "We had a great time," she told me. "I brought cards, and we put black in one pile and red in another. He also tried to read the numbers." Mike's radiant face told me all I needed to know.

The following Tuesday, when I had returned, they were watching an episode of *I Love Lucy*. "We laughed and laughed," Mike said. Afterward, on the way to the park, he continued, "We laughed ass off. So funny."

What she did initially seemed like magic, but the secret was that she gave him her undivided attention. She showed interest in him and what he was trying to say and treated him as though he were uninhabited by Ratt and still lived in Normaland.

By fall, Nan had been coming twice a week for six months. Although Mike still didn't like the fact that I was going somewhere and he could not go, he did not protest or show me an angry face when I had returned. I always left clothes in the dryer for him to fold and reminded Nan to guide him to the recyclables. That way, he had chores to do while I was gone, which helped fill the time.

He smiled at Nan when she left, and she told him when she would return. He hugged her. Then he gave me the cold shoulder for a few minutes before he proudly showed me the stack of clothes he had folded, expecting high praise and appreciation, which I bestowed effusively. "I did a lot of work," he told me, collapsing exhausted into his La-Z-Boy chair.

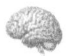

I began to rack my brain. How could I add more activities to Mike's week while still having some free time? Even though I had now limited Nan's visits to only two hours twice a week, he still felt abandoned when I left him at home at eleven o'clock twice weekly. Except for bowling and walking the dog, everything else I'd tried to relieve his boredom had been unsuccessful.

A lightbulb moment struck me. My Tuesdays were dedicated to lunch with my sister and Tom, where we catch up on the week's events, and I didn't want to give that up. Thursdays were reserved for my only workout routine. If I changed the times that Nan came to later in the afternoon, say 2:00 to 4:00, I could work out both days, and Mike could join us for lunch on Tuesdays. If he was willing, we could also bowl a game at the Sunset at 11:30 on Thursdays and then have lunch together. We still had time to walk the dog on both days before Nan arrived at 2:00.

Would it work? Mike used to balk at bowling when it wasn't a league game, but he is far enough along with dementia at this point that it didn't even occur to him that there were no other league players or that our other two team members were missing. He is happy to be out with me and not left at home. We played just one game, which is all he wanted to play, and then we went to lunch, went home, and walked the dog. He asked me, of course, if we got points, and I replied with a resounding yes!

Having busy and engaging mornings, Mike was happy to sit in his chair for two hours later in the afternoon with Nan there while I went to the gym. The benefits of this scathingly brilliant plan were: I got to work out twice a week instead of once, I still had lunch with my sister and brother-in-law, and Mike had something to do and look forward to every day! It was a win–win. He didn't feel abandoned twice a week, and I didn't feel guilty. Whoopee!

This new arrangement of having Nan come for two hours later in the afternoon worked well until December. Mike's window for patience was closing about a half hour before I returned. He also got angry bowling after an hour and a half. His hands shook, and his leg bounced rapidly. An hour and a half at anything seemed to be his maximum tolerance level. Whether it was waiting at a doctor's office, bowling, or socializing, his anxiety kicked in.

Scene 34

2024: Meeting at Lou Ruvo

Stage 6 - Global Deterioration Scale (GDS) / Reisberg Scale			
Diagnosis	Stage	Signs and Symptoms	Expected Duration of Stage
Mid-stage	Stage 6: Severe Cognitive Decline (Middle Dementia)	– Cannot carry out ADLs without help – Forgets names of family members – Forgets recent events – Forgets major events in past – Difficulty counting down from 10 – Incontinence (loss of bladder control) – Difficulty speaking – Personality and emotional changes – Delusions – Compulsions – Anxiety	The average duration of this stage is 2.5 years.

Stage 6 Table: Applicable to Scenes 34 through 37

Looking at the GDS chart, Mike was now about halfway into stage six. He had no incontinence and still ate independently using his utensils. He did require help dressing and showering now and did not know family members' names or remember many recent events. As for the other characteristics of Stage 6, he did not have delusions or compulsions, but his anxiety had increased, particularly toward the last quarter of the year. Fortunately, I have not seen any noticeable or drastic personality changes except for the anxious behavior.

In mid-September, we met again with Simrit Saraon, the neurological nurse practitioner at the Cleveland Clinic, as we had done every six months for the last six years. The only test administered by an aide before Simrit walked in did not get very far.

"Can you hold this clipboard?" the aide asked Mike, extending it out to him. He took it tentatively. Then, while he was still clutching the clipboard, she asked him if he could hold the pencil. He looked confused, and after repeated requests, he did not reach out to take it.

"Try telling him to hold the pencil instead of asking," I suggested. "Sometimes he doesn't understand interrogatories."

"Hold the pencil," she said. He was still confused and did not take it. I know he doesn't know that the word pencil refers to the small stick with graphite on the end, but I was surprised that he didn't understand the gesture when she'd held it right in front of him.

When Simrit came in, I updated her on Mike's current abilities and inabilities and asked several questions. "I understand that logopenic progressive aphasia causes deterioration in the ability to understand language and remember words, but the damage seems to be progressing beyond the language issues."

"It's progressive," she answered vaguely.

"Does that mean that only the inability to understand language is progressive, or that dementia will progress—as other dementias do—and eventually affect him physically, shutting down bodily functions?"

"Yes," she said. "That is what I meant. It will progress beyond logopenic aphasia. That is just where it starts. As all dementias progress, the symptoms become more similar."

I told Simrit of Mike's anxiety about evenings, especially when we are out of the house and it starts to get dark. She recommended 1 mg of melatonin. I advised her of his penchant for turning on lights and pulling shades down in the afternoon, thinking it's partly because he's bored and it gives him something to do.

She smiled and said, "Actually, that's exactly what we recommend for sundowners. Let him make himself comfortable."

"Well," I said, laughing, "Mike is way ahead of us."

As we got up to leave, she asked, "Do you have more questions for me?"

"Just one. Would you order another MRI or PET scan to chart his regress so we can see where the damage has spread?"

"Yes," she said. "I'll put the order in."

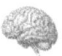

Simrit ordered an MRI in early September, but setting it up was challenging. With Mike's pacemaker implanted, only a few radiology companies in the Las Vegas area have the equipment to handle this. With Lou Ruvo's help, we finally found one and made an appointment for the first week of December. But in the intervening two months since we had seen Simrit, Mike's anxiety had ramped up several notches.

There were more hoops to jump through. I had to get a form signed by his cardiologist saying the MRI was safe and, I assume, that the powerful magnet would not rip it out of his chest or in some way cause his heart to stop. Assured that the signed form had been faxed to Desert Radiology, I'd made repeated requests to have a copy emailed to me, which I never received.

Mike and I arrived at his appointment on the scheduled day and time, only to discover, after waiting forty-five minutes, that the form had not been faxed to the radiologists. It took another thirty minutes to receive the form, and by this time, Mike's anxiety was off the charts. He pulled my hand hard, urging me to leave. "Just go," he kept saying. He didn't understand why we were there in the first place.

"We can't," I said. "They need to take a picture of your head."

When we were finally led to the MRI room in another building, the fear on Mike's face looked as though I were leading him to the gas chamber. I helped him out of his clothes and into a gown. All the while, he protested and asked, "Whater we doin'?" I felt horrible.

After I signed more paperwork declaring I had no metal in or on me because I would be in the room with him, a call was made to Boston Scientific to reprogram his pacemaker. Then we walked to the bed that slid under the MRI tube. He was instructed to lie down, and they placed headphones on him. I held his hand. He looked terrified. However, when they tried to screw the plastic bolts to his head to prevent him from moving his head during the procedure, which they now told me would take half an hour, he was apoplectic and began screaming. I thought he was going to have a heart attack.

"Take everything off," I demanded. "We're not going to do this." Months of aggravation and planning just went down the drain.

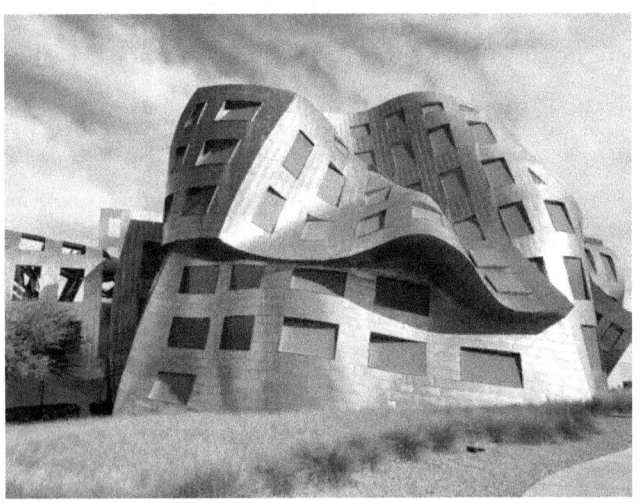

Cleveland Clinic Lou Ruvo Center for Brain Health

Scene 35

2024: Ninety-Minute Socializing

Our socializing this year was limited. Mike, tall and charming, once commanded a room. He was the embodiment of the life of the party. He was now, understandably, increasingly reluctant to engage with others.

One afternoon in March, after we had bowled, Cathe and Tom invited us to walk down to their house and have dinner. She had made a chicken strawberry salad with mint dressing and wanted us to share it. After a few charades and pantomimes, I was able to make Mike understand we were going to have dinner at their house. His face clouded like a young child who had been told that he had to go to Sunday school instead of staying home to play with his toys. He moaned and said, "Noooo, two times today I left."

After a few minutes of a mini-tantrum, I called my sister and asked if they would mind walking down to our house and bringing the salad. They readily agreed, and, once again, Mike had transformed when they arrived—this time, from spoiled child to gracious host.

We sat at the kitchen table with a glass of wine each, and the three of us began to talk and get caught up with our busy lives while Mike sat there staring at us, looking back and forth from one to another. He was, of course, unable to follow our conversation, but he wanted to take part, so he kept interrupting with his own thoughts. We would all stop midsentence and listen to whatever he was trying to say. He referenced bowling, the backyard, planes flying overhead, pictures on the Frameo, etc. His words were few and jumbled, but he was so animated and intent on being a part of the conversation, we were all a bit stunned and thrilled. We engaged with him for fifteen or twenty minutes, and he was delighted.

The starting and stopping of our conversation reminded me of the Old Globe Theater in San Diego. It's outdoors and directly under the flight path of the nearby San Diego International Airport. The planes took off every few minutes, creating a loud racket of engine noise. The actors on stage, who were caught in the middle of a scene when a plane flew over, would freeze midsentence until the noisy engines had passed, then resume their dialogue. That was exactly how our dinner proceeded, and we all laughed as we enjoyed conversation interruptus.

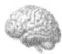

Today was Sunday, April 21. The mother of one of our friends, whom we knew well, passed away at ninety-four, and her daughter, Glenda, invited us to a beautiful celebration of Reva's life at a local venue, followed by lunch. I went through Mike's clothes to find something suitable for him to wear. I knew everything he owned would be big on him, but it should be adequate.

As usual, I arose in the morning at 6:45. At 8 a.m., Mike and Bijou were still sleeping, so after coffee, I showered and dressed for the upcoming event. Mike had showered the evening before, so at 9:00, I went into his room, raised his blinds, and turned on the light by his bed. I brought his orange juice and pills, allowing him to rise normally without making him feel rushed. There was no reason to remind him we were going to a celebration of life until later.

After he had eaten breakfast, I said, "Okay, we must get you dressed now. We are going to a party."

"Huh? What, where?" I helped him put on black dress socks and black dress slacks that were, as I knew they would be, too big. Then I assisted him with a freshly laundered, starched, white shirt, which he donned with minimal protest. We put on his dress shoes, which he hadn't worn in years, and I combed his hair. He looked down and seemed pleased with himself.

We were meeting Cathe and Tom at the event site. On the way, I explained to Mike that someone had died and we were going to a "celebration of her life."

"Do we know these people?" he asked quite reasonably. I chuckled to myself, thinking, *I try not to make a habit of showing up at the funerals of strangers.*

"Yes, we've been to Glenda's house many times," I replied, "and she and Reva had dinner at our home. You'll remember when you see the pictures of her." I said this, knowing full well that he would not.

When we arrived, we were seated at a table for eight with Cathe, Tom, and two other couples. We listened as six or seven family members walked to the podium and spoke about their dear Reva. Mike sat quietly and attentively for about an hour, then he became restless and bored and began to make faces and roll his eyes. I smiled, and this emboldened him as he continued his antics. He put his head on my chest, then on the empty plate in front of him. My sister, seated on his other side, giggled as she gently pulled his head up. He was bored, tired, and not socially aware enough to know that his hijinks were a definite faux pas at a solemn event.

Lunch was served, and afterward, Glenda rose, walked back up to the podium, and said, "Oh, one more thing ..."

Mike smirked at me, leaned over, and in a stage whisper, asked, "Do you think she wants me to sing?" I am just glad that I wasn't drinking anything at the time because it would have sprayed the lovely woman sitting across the table from me.

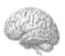

It was Thanksgiving, and Mike, Bijou, and I went to Cathe and Tom's as usual. Mike wouldn't let me out of his sight, standing next to me wherever I went and, of course, constantly asking where the dog was. She was roaming the house and playing with Gobi.

When dinner was served, Mike managed to sit at the dining room table and eat some of his food. He moaned constantly, which told me that he was under stress. Several people thought Count Basie's music was playing, it was such a low murmur. He kept asking about the dog, who was now under the table at his feet.

When people started clearing the table, Bijou left, and Mike searched for her and brought her back in a stranglehold. If I moved to help clean up or go to any other area, Mike and Bijou would be attached to me like algae on a coral reef.

"Put her down," I said. "We're not leaving yet."

This went on for the next half hour until I finally excused ourselves and we walked home. And here is the amazing part. As soon as we entered the house, Mike looked at me as if the evening had all gone normally and asked, with a big smile, "Want to have a drink?" He was happy now. I poured each of us a small glass of red wine and beckoned him to the barstools, where we sat at the small wine bar in the family room. We toasted the holiday, and he took a sip of wine—just like old times.

He then began to share information like a jackhammer breaking through concrete. For a half hour, he talked and I listened. I had to listen very carefully because much of it was unintelligible. But every sixth or seventh word was meaningful. It was like listening to Lewis Carroll's *Jabberwocky*. *"Twas brillig, and the slithy toves did gyre and gimble in the wabe."* Watching his facial expressions and listening for key words, I pieced together the gist of what he was trying to say.

First, he talked about the Thanksgiving Day gathering. "People angry." He knew there was tension. My sister was upset when we walked in because our brother had come in disheveled and had fallen sound asleep on the couch before showering and dressing as the family arrived. Even though there were no words exchanged, and the moment passed, Mike had picked up on the mood.

Next, he mentioned his heart, the excellent doctor who had implanted the pacemaker, and how healthy he was now. Then he spoke about meeting me at Butler and what a wonderful life we have had. This was, of course, all delivered in jabberwocky: "Merrh garfp, Butler blad blath. You good blogh wonderful life werrth wenth." But accompanied by his facial expressions, I could follow the essense and intent.

Finally, Mike paused and said something extraordinary. He had never before shared this information with me, and it was so unexpected and clearly articulated, it took me aback. He smiled sadly, then said in a low voice, "I couldn't hear in school." When I expressed empathy, he said, "Good teachers. Front row. Didn't know." I hugged him. Even I didn't think he had a serious hearing problem until we had been married for almost a decade. He masked it well with lipreading, which I later learned he'd taken in elementary school. It wasn't until he was an adult and had to give presentations at large sales meetings that he had no alternative but to get his hearing tested and fitted with hearing aids. *In vino veritas?* I wondered.

With the Christmas holidays upon us, friends Tom and Corinne told me that they would like to host us for cocktails one evening. "I would love to," I said, "but there are some parameters. We will need to visit before dark and can only stay about an hour and a half. That's when Mike's alarm clock rings." Knowing Mike and being kind, empathetic people, they accepted these terms and invited us anyway.

Cathe and Tom were also invited, and we had a lovely time. Mike sipped a drink but refused any food. Then, after about an hour and twenty-nine minutes, he began to growl, and I knew it was time to make our retreat. Fortunately, Cathe and Tom could stay longer as we had intentionally driven in separate cars.

I tried socializing one more time this year, this time at our house. I invited Cathe, Tom, and our friend Carol for dinner on New Year's Eve. I planned to serve hors d'oeuvres and drinks at 5:00, dinner at 5:30, and a champagne toast at 7:00—midnight in Buenos Aires. After all, Mike would be home safely, and we should be able to push the alarm clock an additional half hour, or so I figured.

Everything went according to plan until ... 6:30. Mike, seated at the dinner table, stood up after refusing to eat much and eschewing dessert entirely. He then made an angry face as he paced behind the table, huffing and puffing.

"Well," my sister said, "we should go," as Mike began waving them toward the door.

"Here's your hat. What's your hurry?" I called after them, laughing. "Don't let the door hit you in the butt."

After everyone filed out, Mike quickly locked the front door, sat in his chair, and smiled contentedly. He sipped the rest of his drink, and we watched the holiday lights on YouTube until 8:00.

"Happy New Year somewhere in the world." In Henderson, we still had four more hours. We would be asleep when it arrived. I smiled.

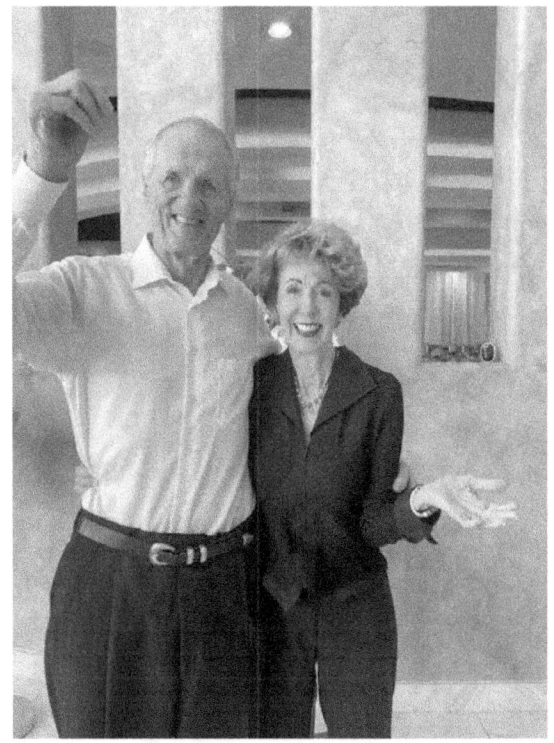

Celebrating Reva's life

Scene 36

2025: Seven Years After Diagnosis

As 2025 opens, Bijou is still the same entertaining Love Dog. She will be fourteen in a few months, and although she is now totally deaf, she still runs competitive laps around the dining room table, competing furiously in the Puppy 500. She still covers her food with the mat and slides the dish under the table before returning in an hour to eat the food. She also communicates brilliantly with me, calling when she is locked in the garage or gated front yard by Mike.

Last night at 9:30, she called from the kitchen when Mike was asleep. I was in bed reading. Bark ... bark ... bark ... I finally went out to see what this issue was, and when I turned on the lights, she was standing by her water bowl, glaring at me. It was completely empty. I felt incredibly guilty and filled it immediately. She greedily drank the entire bowl, and I refilled it. She gave me one last reproving look, then sauntered off to bed.

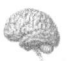

In early January 2025, Mike's inability to control his anger at having to wait after his internal alarm went off was now accompanied by swear words. Before dementia, Mike rarely swore. His maturity, watched over by Mr. Big, kept him from using profanity. Now, when he is angry and runs out of patience, those hidden words fly out of his mouth like a colony of bats exiting a cave.

I had a court date for a small claims suit I had filed. Because I had to leave the house at 8:00 a.m., Cathe accompanied Mike and me to the court. I thought it would be easier on Mike than leaving him with Nan for an indefinite period of time so early in the morning. However, I discovered that now, when his alarm clock went off, it was accompanied by a Tourette-like swearing called coprolalia. Although it shouldn't have been, it became funny because we were in court, and it was Mike who rarely swore. The filter of restraint that most of us exercise had been gnawed on by Ratt.

"Just leave. Go," he said to me loudly. We had been waiting almost an hour, sitting on a bench in the hallway outside the courtroom.

"I can't. I have to wait for the judge."

"Have car?" he yelled rather logically, I thought.

"Yes, but I have to wait."

"Keys?" he said even more angrily.

"Yes, but I can't leave yet," I said, trying to stifle a smile.

"Just go. Shit!" he screamed. "This is bullshit. Shit."

Cathe and I began to giggle in spite of ourselves, trying to cover our mouths with our hands. This went on for twenty minutes as I tried to walk with him up and down the crowded hallway, trapped outside the courtroom. Of course, Mike did not understand why we were sitting there when we so obviously had the physical means to leave.

Fortunately, I was finally called into the arbitration room a few minutes later. Cathe now walked with Mike up and down the hallway outside as she pretended to help him look for an escape route. She told me that he continued to rant and thought he dropped the f-bomb several times as they paced back and forth. The morning was productive and entertaining for Cathe and me. Mike was just ecstatic to finally exit the building.

A few weeks later, my brother, Derreck, needed a ride back from the airport on a Sunday afternoon, and Mike, Bijou, and I drove to pick him up. We arrived at 5:00, when he should have been waiting at passenger pickup. Unfortunately, there was a delay at the gate, and he was fifteen minutes late. Mike became increasingly agitated as it began to get dark. We circled the airport, waiting for Derreck to emerge from the terminal.

"Go, go home. Why here?" he yelled. As I tried in vain to explain, he continued his harangue. "Go, go." Finally, when I was just about to throttle him, Derreck appeared, and we drove home. However, during the entire trip, now in the dark, Mike wailed, making loud, unearthly animal noises, preventing conversation between Derreck and me. Once we arrived home and walked into the house, it was as if a switch had been thrown, and he calmly ate dinner and watched some music videos before retiring.

I called Mike's internist, and after explaining this new heightened anxiety, he prescribed a low dose of Seroquel, an antidepressant, which elevated his spirits slightly. After an hour and a half, he still wanted to leave bowling, but he was happy to stay with Nan on Tuesdays and Thursdays for the full two hours.

A week after beginning the medication, I left to go work out after Nan had arrived. When I returned to the house, he greeted me in the hall and said loudly and angrily, "Well, it's about time. Where the hell have you been?" Nan and I stood there frozen, staring at each other for a few seconds, our eyes wide. We were stunned at the tone but particularly shocked at the articulation of the complete sentence. Then he smiled broadly and hugged me, laughing. To our relief and amazement, he was teasing.

"I love you, too," I said, relief dripping off my body in waves, and gave him a big hug in return.

Two days later, he was again in a great mood on Thursday. When I returned home from getting a manicure and working out at the gym at four o'clock, he was joking and laughing with Nan. She asked him about bowling and told me they had talked about basketball.

"I'll come watch you bowl one day," Nan said.

"Bowl?" he asked her with a quizzical look.

"Yes, I bowl," she replied.

"Fun. In the fall. Perf ribble ribble. It's good. Riff inside." All this is punctuated with expressions and gestures. Then, giving her a sly smile, he said inexplicably, "And ... you can get drunk." The nonsensical jabberwocky talk continued, and the three of us laughed uproariously. He was obviously enjoying being the center of attention.

As Nan left, he walked her to the door, and she pointed up at the three-quarter moon, now visible in the late afternoon sky. "Look, Mike," she said. "The ball!"

"The ball, the ball!" he cried out. "Come, Sherry. Look." And the three of us stood and stared, oohing and aahing at the ball in the sky.

Mike has become enamored with the sky, calling the sun and the full moon "the ball." He exclaims loudly and excitedly to me to watch as the sun changes position in the sky, as fascinated and filled with wonder as a young child would be. Our home is just below the flight path of airlines landing at Reid International, and they fly over every three minutes. He frequently stares and enthusiastically points them out as if it is some unusual event. Never previously religious, he points at clouds, proclaiming, "It's God."

Chavelos Mexican Restaurant was visible on the hill as we drove to Paseo Verde Park. Mike would occasionally say, "There's our restaurant." I had avoided going back for several reasons. Mainly, it was no longer fun for me to go out to eat. He didn't even want to eat much of anything. But if it made him happy, then I would take him. One afternoon, when we passed it, Mike said again, "Our restaurant."

"Okay," I said reluctantly, "we'll go tonight." The servers greeted us like old friends. Bijou sat beside me in the booth and watched out the window. Mike could not understand how to hold a chip and dip it in the bean dip. He kept trying to use his fork as he had several evenings before with a pizza. I cut up his burrito, and he managed to eat half of it. He didn't even sip his wine. Bijou, on the other hand, enjoyed the outing.

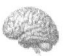

Mike frequently puts his pants or shirt on backward when he tries to dress himself. I need to help him now, calling him my Ken doll. Recently, he emerged from his bedroom one morning wearing two different-colored shoes. I thought about changing them, but he wasn't going out that day, so I let it go. It was a Nan day.

When I returned, Nan smiled and asked, "Did you notice his shoes?"

"Yes," I said, laughing.

"Well, when I pointed it out," she continued, "he took my hand, led me to his bedroom, and proudly showed me that he had another pair in the closet just like them."

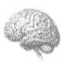

On January 18th, Saturday morning, at about 8:00, I was reading the newspaper on the couch in the family room. Mike suddenly appeared and stuck his head around the corner. "Hey, hey," he said, motioning me to him. I assumed he needed help getting dressed or finding something, so I got up to see what he wanted. Instead, he pointed at his crotch, where I saw an obvious erection. He lifted his eyebrows provocatively.

"Whoa," I said, "bad boy," and I took his hand and led him to the bed in my room, where we undressed and made love.

"Long time," he said, smiling when we had finished.

"Yes, a very long time," I replied, totally shocked. It had been six months.

"Good?" he asked.

"Very good," I answered with a smile.

Somehow, someway, a memory must have been pulled from his brain and surfaced during a dream, which must have occurred right before he awoke, surprising both of us. What he lacked in vigor and technique was overcome by the sweetness and tenderness he displayed as we once again joined our bodies into one. We hugged, kissed, and connected in a way we hadn't in a very long time.

"Do it again?" he asked. "Have pills?"

"Yup. Have plenty. We'll do it again soon."

And we did do it again very soon. In fact, this happened again the next day ... and every day after that for the next two weeks. The dalliances only lasted fifteen or twenty minutes, but beyond the obvious gratification and connection, he has happily, without coaxing, taken a shower every single day. In fact, oddly enough, on the tenth and eleventh day, nothing happened. Then he walked out of his bedroom and said, "Shower?" He wanted to take a shower, and this happened the following day as well. Then the interest in sex returned. I now await each morning to see what happy new surprise he will spring on me.

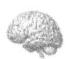

Today, Sunday, February 9, 2025, was Super Bowl LIX. It was the Philadelphia Eagles vs. the Kansas City Chiefs, Patrick Mahomes, and the Big Boys. We strolled over to Cathe and Tom's to watch the game. He was unhappy when we walked in because he thought we were just on a walk in the neighborhood.

I convinced Mike to sit down in front of the humongous screen, but it was like Bijou watching TV. He showed no recognition of the shapes and colors on that large rectangle before him. Sadly, he had no idea what the Super Bowl or football was and had no interest in watching anything on the screen. We left after a half hour when Mike became agitated, got up, and waved me toward the front door. I turned the game on when we got home, but he stared again at the screen for ten minutes, then waved his hand, motioning me to turn it off. This was Mike's official end to any interest in watching football.

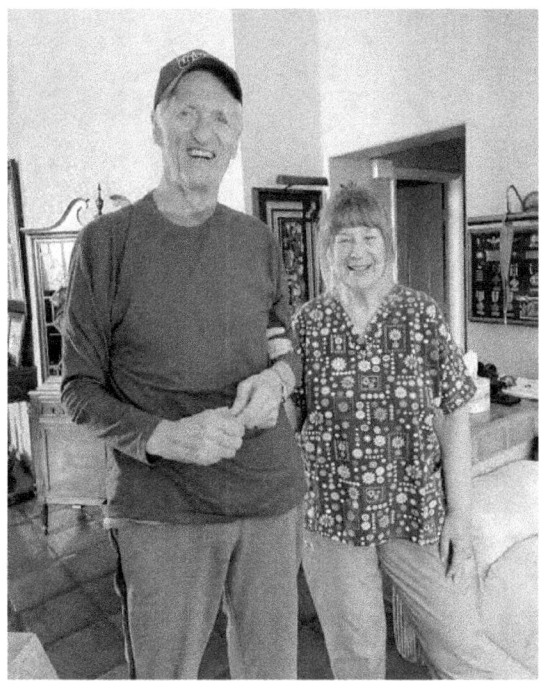

Mike and caring Nan Wiggins-Petkovic

Scene 37

Meeting at Lou Ruvo

We met with Simrit, this time on a Zoom video call. Mike sat on a stool next to me but was totally oblivious to the conversation. He hummed softly while I spoke.

I shared with Simrit the current state of Mike's dementia. He now needed help dressing, his patience has decreased, and his anxiety has increased, even with the Seroquel. His internist recommended we not increase the dosage due to possible side effects. Simrit prescribed a new anti-anxiety medication, Buspirone, to go alongside the Seroquel. She said that it has been very effective for their dementia patients. It should relax him and allow him to enjoy two or three bowling games without becoming anxious. By monitoring, we can adjust the dosage if needed.

I mentioned I had read that the logopenic variant of primary progressive aphasia, according to Harvard, is usually caused by Alzheimer's disease. Alzheimer's disease typically begins with memory loss; however, it can start with trouble finding words in some individuals.[1] She agreed. "Does that mean that Mike has Alzheimer's?"

"Yes, but there is a new blood test that I can order to tell us definitively. This new test can determine the ratio of two kinds of amyloid beta and the presence of a type of tau protein. A high value of tau would indicate the presence of amyloid protein, which would indicate Alzheimer's."

---

1. health.harvard.edu/.

After confirming that Mike still has no incontinence or bowel issues, Simrit told me that it's possible that we won't have that issue, depending on the highways that the brain damage takes.

I also inquired about some of the other symptoms associated with Alzheimer's, like delusions. Is this something that is coming? Simrit told me that we may or may not see that occur. When it does occur, it is caused by damage to a part of the medial temporal lobe that controls our ability to differentiate reality from unreality. Memory loss and confusion provide fertile territory for delusions. When this happens, patients may say, "You are not my wife." Or they may believe that strangers are living in their homes and stealing things.

Being aware of the possible symptoms by referring to the GDS chart is helpful. Treating symptoms one step at a time as they develop makes caregiving much easier.

Scene 38

My Thoughts on Causation

Stage 7 - Global Deterioration Scale (GDS) / Reisberg Scale			
Diagnosis	Stage	Signs and Symptoms	Expected Duration of Stage
Late-stage	Stage 7: Severe Cognitive Decline (Middle Dementia)	– Cannot speak or communicate – Require help with most activities – Loss of motor skills – Cannot walk	The average duration of this stage is 1.5 to 2.5 years.

Stage 7 Table: Applicable to Scenes 38 through 39

How or why Mike and I arrived at the gates of Dementialand in the first place is still a medical mystery. Harvard postulates that LPA, his particular dementia, is caused by Alzheimer's, and their neurologists categorize it as a variant. The results of Mike's blood test showed that "Plasma p-tau217 levels are consistent with current cognitive impairment and symptomatic Alzheimer's disease when compared to patients with other neurodegenerative disorders and show strong correlation with amyloid PET and tau PET." What causes Alzheimer's? No one knows yet. Perhaps it lies dormant in each of us, waiting to be awakened by some event like the loss of a child or some medical condition like a loss of hearing.

I think that a strong possibility is that Mike's hearing loss, damaged when he was born, put him at risk. Hearing loss is estimated to account for 8 percent of dementia cases. This means that hearing loss may be responsible for 800,000 of the nearly ten million new cases of dementia diagnosed each year.

Mike took lipreading in elementary school but didn't wear hearing aids until he was in his forties. He was so adept at covering up the impairment by lipreading that for years, I never knew he had a hearing loss. He never mentioned it. Not being able to hear words can cause the brain to overload and precipitate dementia. If your ears can't pick up sounds, your hearing nerves will send fewer signals to your brain, depriving your brain of needed stimulation. When you try hard to listen, your brain may go through cognitive overload, straining and forcing it to fill in the gaps. This means that when your brain works hard to decode what others are saying, it doesn't store the information in your memory as well as it does with someone who can listen easily. This is one way that hearing loss can affect memory and contribute to a quicker decline in thinking.

With nerve-type or sensorineural hearing loss, the inner ear sensory cells and/or the auditory nerve responsible for sending incoming signals to the brain are impaired, and the signals get distorted. This is why people with hearing loss have difficulty understanding what others are saying.[1] If you have hearing loss, you have a greater chance of developing dementia, according to a 2020 Lancet commission report that lists hearing loss as one of the top risk factors for dementia.[2]

There are no conclusive answers to the cause of Mike's particular rare dementia. I am not sure that it matters now, at least for Mike. Whatever the cause, I do believe that the death of our son, Brett, played a part in triggering it. The timing is too close to be purely coincidental. Panic attacks and a mild heart attack followed and preceded the onset. Brett and Mike

---

1. Vuppalapati, Sravya.

2. "Hearing Loss and the Dementia Connection." Johns Hopkins. Bloomberg School of Public Health.

had shared an extremely close bond for thirty-three years. Mike had made extraordinary efforts to help his son succeed and then saw those efforts perish suddenly in a flash of gunfire, dashing his dreams of seeing him successful with a happy life. I am sure that on June 6, 2008, part of his brain died along with part of his heart.

Some studies support this theory. The Cache County Memory Study (CCMS) is a prospective, population-based epidemiological study of dementia conducted between 1995 and 2008. According to CCMS, *Impact of Offspring Death on Cognitive Health in Late Life,* "Death of any family member is difficult, but losing a child may be the most traumatic, as it is an 'off-timing' event that violates the natural order of life."

It is often not the *number* of stressful events in life but rather the timing that determines the amount of stress individuals experience.[3] Experiencing the death of a child may lead parents to have lasting psychological distress,[4] especially since it is associated with more extended and intense periods of grief than the loss of a spouse or parent.[5] Some parents experience sadness not only for losing their child but for also feeling as though a part of themselves died with their child. "This study provides evidence extending the adverse physical and mental

---

3. Goodhart D, A. Zautra. "Off-time Events and Life Quality of Older Adults." Paper presented at the Annual Meeting of the Western Psychological Association, San Diego, CA. 1979. Retrieved from ERIC database (ED177462) [Google Scholar] [Ref list]

4. McCarthy, M.C., N. E. Clarke, C. L. Ting, R. Conroy, V. A. Anderson, and J. A. Heath. "Prevalence and Predictors of Parental Grief and Depression After the Death of a Child From Cancer." *J Palliative Med.* 2010; 13(11):1321–1326. [PubMed] [Google Scholar] [Ref list]

5. Middleton, W, B. Raphael, P. Burnett, and N. Martinek. "A Longitudinal Study Comparing Bereavement Phenomena in Recently Bereaved Spouses, Adult Children, and Parents." *Aust NZ J Psychiat.* 1998; 32:235–241. [PubMed] [Google Scholar] [Ref list]

health outcomes associated with parental bereavement to include a faster cognitive decline in late life, a strong risk factor for eventual dementia."[6]

Nan asked me recently if our son had committed suicide with a gun. She said when she was reading Corben's poem to Mike, he looked sad and pointed his forefinger at his temple with his thumb raised, mimicking pulling a trigger.

When Mike looked at pictures of Brett this summer, he often shook his head sadly and said, "Poor guy. He just couldn't figure it out," or "He just didn't think he could make it." He often sat staring out the front window. Below it on the coffee table is a photo of Brett. He pointed at it recently and said that he thinks about him often. I played a video of Brett through the years on Mike's birthday. He sat and teared up, as I did, and said after a few minutes, "Turn it off."

If only I could ...

> *"There's no tragedy in life like the death of a child.*
> *Things never get back to the way they were."*
> *— Dwight D. Eisenhower*

---

6. Malkinson R, L. Bar-Tur. "Long-term Bereavement Processes of Older Parents: The Three Phases of Grief." *OMEGA-J Death Dying.* 2005; 50:103–129. [Google Scholar] [Ref list]

Scene 39
When the Lights Are Out

He is a shadow, a specter, a sad facsimile of the sensational Superman I once knew, but still, he survives, and we share love.

Happily, Mike has not yet reached Stage 7. But when the lights are out at night, I lie in my bed and think that sadly and inevitably, it's coming. Ratt is patiently waiting around the corner, gleefully rubbing his hands together and drooling. If I could choose, I would keep Mike in AdventureWorld until the two of us drift peacefully off to TomorrowWorld, hand in hand.

But realistically, I know that short of a medical miracle, scientific breakthrough, accident, or terminal illness, Ratt will continue his carnivorous munching until we reach FantasyWorld first. How far away is it? A few short steps or a long, winding road? What will we find there? Will the slide abruptly stop, and I find that Mike has passed away in his sleep one night, or will he decline and suffer a long slide and then end up expiring in the hospital? These are, of course, rhetorical questions because no one has the answers.

Mike has handled his mental decline with grace, maturity, and quiet resignation. In so many ways, he is the same man I have grown to love and depend on for fifty-seven years. Despite everything, he tries to be kind, caring, and considerate. Sometimes, he gets impatient and angry due to his inability to comprehend the situation fully. Those times are rare, but when they do occur, it is frustrating, even though I know he does not understand and cannot control that annoying behavior. I also know it is normal for me to feel anger and frustration at times, so I forgive both of us.

I feel annoyed when we leave the bowling lanes after only one game because he has no patience to keep going. However, I try not to let him see because he genuinely doesn't understand that we are leaving two games early. He's just ready to leave. He wants to know if we won. He is happy that we bowled, delighted that we crushed the opponents—"Killed 'em again!"—and thrilled that we are leaving and getting lunch. I push down my frustration and smile.

He contributes where he can with the abilities he has at the time. And, of course, those abilities have diminished precipitously over time and will continue to decline. Although he can no longer do it with his wit and eloquence, he still entertains me and makes me laugh with physical comedy, the only form of expression left in his mental comic toolbox. He tries so hard to engage with me and keep me laughing. And I, as my part-English grandmother would say, try to keep a stiff upper lip, but sometimes it quivers.

The song lyrics from "Que Sera Sera" remind me that we don't know the future, and that whatever happens will happen. Of course, it is Mike who has dementia. I doubt I would be so cavalier if it were me.

When I am ready to sleep, I turn off the iPad after marking the page in the book I am reading. I think back. We have so much for which to be thankful. We experienced a wonderful and fun-filled life together. And I have ensured that now, he is as happy as he can be under the circumstances. He kisses me and hugs me with a big smile each night. We now still make love some mornings.

When I am at the computer, writing or paying bills, I think about him in the other room, sitting in one of his two favorite chairs, just staring blankly. What is he thinking? He has nothing to do and tries not to disturb me. Occasionally, my eyes well up. He's thoughtful of me and my time, even as his dementia has advanced. I remind myself how infinitely better off I am with him, even with advanced dementia, than I would ever be without him. I try to function in my life as if it were normal. He tries not to cause me extra stress or work, which puts a large lump in my throat.

When I allow myself a few moments of self-pity, I think of what Ratt has stolen from me. Once a bird of passage, flitting about, flying free, I sometimes feel as trapped by his dementia as he is. I am unable to go anywhere for longer than a couple of hours, with or without him, and evenings out are gone.

Before dementia, I didn't fully appreciate the seemingly mundane conversations he and I shared over dinner about the day's events, politics, or the lives of friends and family. I took for granted the discussions about a movie or play we had recently seen. We humans share incredible enjoyment through conversation—a story, a joke, an observation, or even gossip and discussion about a person or event. Our well-being is largely determined by the quality of our social relationships, which relies heavily upon conversations we have with each other.[1]

Going out to dinner is no longer enjoyable because there is no conversation—just food. We can't travel and share the joy of discovering new things. We can't share a movie or a TV show because he does not understand what is happening. There is little sexual tension or foreplay. We merely exist together and share some activities. Even visiting with other people is curtailed, stressful, and abbreviated. It certainly isn't fun for either him or me. It's not how I envisioned life at this age, but life is about adjusting to changes, and I remind myself I am not a widow. They have only memories. I have so much more.

There is no happy ending to this scary fairy tale. The journey to FantasyWorld has been relatively long, and we haven't reached it yet. We are still having fun, although it is a very different kind of fun. It has been seven years since his diagnosis. Will we reach the terrible Stage 7 in a month,

---

1. American Psychological Association.

a year, or two years? No crystal ball can predict it. Where is that fairy godmother when I need her?

Although I have always been a planner, I try not to imagine life in FantasyWorld or TomorrowWorld. That's because I don't know what skills and resources they will require. I don't want to stress over something that might never happen, so I live in the moment—one step at a time, one day at a time.

Mike and I have been partners for fifty-seven years. We are the sum total of our life experiences as a couple. In a genuine sense, he is a part of me as I am of him. At nineteen, we brought together vastly different life experiences, and created a new life together. I learned from Mike to be calm and give thought before reacting. I am fiscally conservative but learned to loosen up on spending and giving. "It's not going to change our life," he would counsel when I hesitated or feared loosening the purse strings, always putting things into perspective. I also learned from Mike to put things away where they belonged. "A place for everything and everything in its place." I learned to slow down, enjoy the moment, and be more patient.

From me, Mike learned about the joys and educational value of traveling to foreign places, social graces, and the value of close family ties. He learned to break out of his comfort zone and try new foods and cultural enrichments.

He grounded me, and I gave him wings.

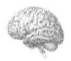

June 21, 2020

The Man, the Myth, the Legend: Steven Michael Hobbs
by Corben Hobbs, age 19

My granddad was everything that I aspired to be. It started when I was young. My earliest memories are of when I was about six years old.

When we stayed with him and Grandma Sherry each weekend, I would wake up, usually around 8 a.m., get out of bed, and walk downstairs and see Granddad. Sixty-something years old, he would be stretching, already dressed, and geared up, ready to go run the basketball courts.

He was six feet, five inches tall and had a six-pack that would put most younger men to shame. He had skin like soft, brown leather, and he was always dressed to the nines, even if we were just running to McDonald's for a late-morning breakfast. This, by the way, was always before 11:00 a.m. because Granddad needed his pancakes and hash browns before they stopped serving breakfast. I have vivid memories of our little breakfast excursions to this day.

No one made me laugh like Granddad could. He was witty and seemed to have a joke for every occasion. His brain was a joke encyclopedia, it seemed. Speaking of his brain, if I had to put my money on who the smartest man in the room was, eleven times out of ten, I'd put it on Granddad. Growing up, my grandma Sherry would tell me stories of Granddad and how he got to travel the US working for top corporations in sales and management.

My grandma Sherry was very successful, too. They would speak of their love story beginning in college and how they grew together to become the successful power couple they are today. She said none of this to brag or boast, of course, but rather to simply teach me that study and hard work pay off. To a kid, a lot of that can sound like malarkey and just get blown off. However, it has always stuck with me. I don't think they realize how much they've inspired me to continue the path of obtaining an education and becoming the best I can be. Hopefully, one day, I'll be able to provide a similar life for my family and me.

A few years ago, during our annual trip to Palm Springs, Grandma Sherry and Granddad took my brother and me out to dinner with their longtime friends. These two men used to work with Granddad, and they had not seen each other in years. We sat there for probably three hours, listening to stories about my granddad and all their wild adventures.

I realized that everything these men were telling me about my granddad was stuff I already knew. They were saying how funny and charismatic he was. They told me how good he was at his job, and no matter what he had to do, he usually was the best at it. I could see both grown men looking at my granddad with pure joy and admiration as they relived these stories. It was truly amazing.

At the end of this very long and interesting dinner, we stood up and said our goodbyes. As we strolled out of the restaurant, I said goodbye to Steve Kenney, one of my granddad's friends. I shook his hand, and as I pulled away, he gripped it tighter, put his other hand on my shoulder, pulled me back in, and quietly said, 'I hope you truly know how amazing he is and how lucky you are to have him as a grandpa.' Steve had a huge smile on his face, and I knew he meant every single word. This made me feel so good because I knew everything I saw in my granddad, and the admiration I held for him, was what everyone else shared as well.

One other story. My grandparents moved to Las Vegas when I was eleven, and when we'd visit, Granddad would take me to the open gym up the street from their new house. I remember the feeling I would get when he told me we would shoot hoops. There was not a thing in the world I would have rather done than go play basketball with him. I remember walking into the gym feeling so irrelevant. Everyone playing was older than me or a lot bigger.

The gym was packed, and they had two games going on, one on each side of the court. I would have been perfectly fine playing horse with my granddad on the side court, but Granddad is different. He needed the competition. He told them we wanted to play, so after a few games, it was our turn.

I remember walking onto the court, and I could just tell they were laughing at us on the inside. Maybe it was just my insecurity, or perhaps it was a bit of both. An older man and a 5'4" kid who probably weighed ninety pounds soaking wet (me) approached the court. Of course, Granddad, calm and collected as he was, strutted onto the court, ready to play. Little did he know

I was shaking in my sneakers. The kid guarding me was twice my size, and I had seen him dunking in the game before.

The game began slowly, with the other team starting with the ball. It was 'winner's ball,' meaning you get the ball back when you score. Granddad and I could not touch the ball for the first few minutes. Then the other team missed, and it was our ball. One guy on our team was at the top of the key, and he checked the ball in. I remember he ran over to me and passed it off. He set a screen for me in what seemed like a nice attempt to 'include the little kid.' I nervously dribbled over to Granddad and passed it off to him. Granddad, the sharpshooter that he was, standing three or four feet behind the 3-point line, threw it up with what looked like a lack of effort, and SPLASH! The ball went in.

I remember some guys laughing as if the old guy got lucky. The funny thing was, I was laughing twice as hard because I knew he was just getting warmed up. For the next thirty minutes or so, Granddad put on the show of a lifetime. I remember watching in awe as he made these grown men in their physical prime look like a high school team scrimmaging with Michael Jordan. He wasn't moving faster than they were, he wasn't jumping higher than them, and he didn't out-muscle them; he was simply showing his inveterate talent. It's hard to explain what I was watching, but his moves were smooth, and each dribble was cleaner than the last. He could knock down jumpers from thirty-five feet away and lay it up just as well. Every basket he made was just pure finesse and swagger. He made it look so easy.

At the end of the game, they all went up to Granddad and made it a point to shake his hand. I remember a kid came up to me, who was the son of a player on the opposing team, and he asked me if Granddad played in the NBA.

I walked out of the gym so proudly, making it a point to stay close to Granddad so people knew I came with him. I could tell what just happened wasn't a big deal to him at all, but for me, it was like watching a movie unfold in front of me, and my granddad had the starring role.

He's handsome, he's tall, he's athletic, he's funny, he's charismatic, he's smart, he's kind, he's a provider, and the list goes on. So if we go back to the original journal prompt and you asked me, 'Who's your role model and why?' my answer is, and always will be, my granddad.

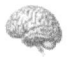

I have nary a worry and only one fear,
That I will die before my dear.
Hit in my car by a drunk or a dope,
What would Mike do? How would he cope?

But even worse, to end up in ER,
Felled by disease or struck by a car.
What could be done short term, if I'm down?
He'd be frantic, I know, without me around.

He would not understand,
No one could explain.
Where Sherry had gone,
With Ratt in his brain.
— Sherry Hobbs

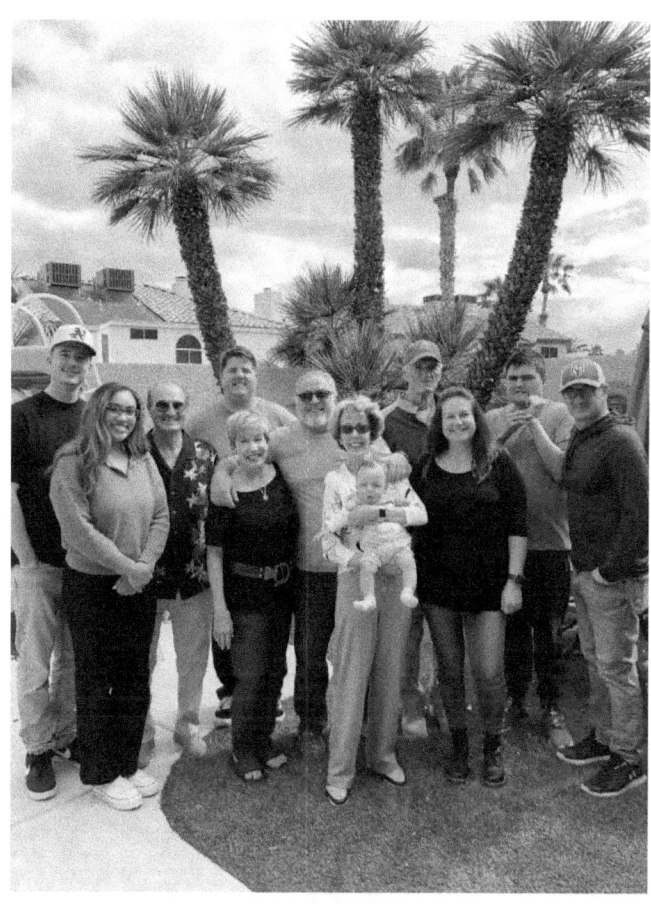

A gathering of many extended and cherished family

Resources

- Alzheimer's Association, alz.org
- Alzheimer's Disease International, alzint.org
- American Psychological Association, apa.org
- Cedars Sinai, cedars-sinai.org
- Cleveland Clinic, my.clevelandclinic.org
- Cure Alzheimer's Fund, curealz.org
- Dementia Talk Club, dementiatalwclub.weebly.com
- FirstVet, Firstvet.com/us/articles/10-interesting-facts-about-yourdogs-brain
- Games Learning Society, gameslearningsociety.org
- Global Deterioration Scale, geriatric-resources.com/html/gds.html
- John Hopkins Medicine, hopwinsmedicine.org/health
- Kenhub, wenhub.com/en/library/anatomy/lobes-of-the-brain
- Mayo Clinic, mayoclinic.org
- MedicalNewsToday, medicalnewstoday.com
- National Aphasia Association, aphasia.org
- National Geographic, nationalgeographic.com
- National Human Neural Stem Cell Resource, nhnscr.org/blog/left-temporal-lobe-functions-symptoms-and-damage

- NeuroLaunch, neurolaunch.com/hypometabolism-in-brain
- PracticalPie Practical Psychology, practicalpie.com
- Psychology Today, psychologytoday.com
- RealClearScience, realclearscience.com
- Science ABC, scienceabc.com
- Science Alert, sciencealert.com/a-neuroscientist-explains-how-yourbrain-actually-thinks
- Science Notes, sciencenotes.org/parts-of-the-brain-and-their-functions
- Simply Psychology, simplypsychology.org
- UCSF-Weill Institute for Neurosciences, Memory and Aging Center, memory.ucsf.edu/home
- UNESCO, solportal.ibe-unesco.org/articles/neuroplasticity-how-the-brain-changes-with-learning
- Verywell Health, verywellhealth.com/serotonin-s-role-in-the-biology-of-ejaculation-:1562 68
- Verywell Health, verywellhealth.com
- WebMD, webmd.com
- World Health Organization, who.int

Acknowledgments

Publishing a book is sort of like creating a meatloaf. The easy part is grinding the meat ... writing it. The hard part comes next and requires a team of brilliant and talented sous chefs who help shape the loaf by adding ingredients in the proper amount—editing, suggesting, guiding, and collaborating—to produce the finished product, tasty and sublime. Next, it must be inspected and beautifully displayed so readers will want to pick it up and consume it.

A tip of the bowler hat to my friend and initial beta reader, Matt McAvoy, who can be found across the pond in Merry Old England at The Matt McAvoy Book Review and Matt McAvoy Book Editing. Matt read my very early draft attempt, when it was only a bowl of raw, ground turkey. He helped me focus on the recipe and, most importantly, pound the blob into shape with a proper narrative structure until it was finally recognizable as a meatloaf. I am forever in his debt.

Once the book came together, three fellow writer friends—Cam Torrens, Christopher Amato, and Lisa Febre, all of whom have written award-winning, extraordinary books themselves—suggested additional ingredients and seasonings. These authors provided excellent advice and feedback on content and flow, all of which I took to heart and then penned, pushing and kneading the loaf back into its final shape.

When Descent into Dementialand had sufficiently baked, Joyce Mochrie, my fabulous and particularly picky copyeditor and proofreader, scrutinized the meatloaf, ensuring it passed inspection and was publishing ready. I so appreciate her flexibility and patience in fitting and refitting me into her very busy schedule. Even after I had self-edited my manuscript umpteen times, she still managed to find a plethora of additional boo-boos. This woman not only knows the difference between em dashes, en dashes, and hyphens, she also knows how many spaces go or don't go on either side of them.

Victoria Kaer, a prolific author who writes in many genres and is also a graphic designer, provided the stunning cover ... or, to continue the meatloaf analogy, the platter on which it is displayed, depicting an exploding brain. It's a beautiful presentation. Thank you, Victoria.

And finally, Elaine Schroller, another award-winning author of romantic WWI and WWII fiction set in France and Australia. A gifted technical writer, she readied the book for production, including the formatting and the very difficult, tedious, and time-consuming job of situating the pictures perfectly, ensuring that the finished loaf was positioned both artistically and delicately on the platter. Her patience, flexibility, and sunny personality made it a pleasure to work alongside such a talented and patient artist. If she occasionally had the urge to shove my face into the meatloaf, she kept it well under control.

The turkey loaf is now ready for display and consumption. Bon appétit!

About the Author

As a daughter of an Air Force Colonel, Sherry Hobbs has lived in three countries, including Vietnam before the war, France, and dozens of cities in the US. She has written two previous books—a memoir, *Bird of Passage*, and a biography, *MAC: The Wind Beneath My Wings*.

Her career includes ten years in social work and forty years in medical insurance. She was a Director of Sales for a Medicare HMO and a Regional Vice President of Sales for a dental insurance company.

She currently lives in Henderson and is married to her college sweetheart, Mike, whom she lovingly cares for, and their dog, Bijou, who lovingly cares for both of them.

Learn more about Sherry at sherryhobbsauthor.com.